Fat in the Fifties

Fat in the Fifties

America's First Obesity Crisis

Nicolas Rasmussen

Johns Hopkins University Press
Baltimore

© 2019 Johns Hopkins University Press
All rights reserved. Published 2019
Printed in the United States of America on acid-free paper

9 8 7 6 5 4 3 2 1

Johns Hopkins University Press
2715 North Charles Street
Baltimore, Maryland 21218-4363
www.press.jhu.edu

Library of Congress Cataloging-in-Publication Data
Names: Rasmussen, Nicolas, 1962– author.
Title: Fat in the fifties : America's first obesity crisis / Nicolas Rasmussen.
Description: Baltimore : Johns Hopkins University Press, [2019] | Includes
bibliographical references and index.
Identifiers: LCCN 2018033818 | ISBN 9781421428710 (hardcover : alk.
paper) | ISBN 1421428717 (hardcover : alk. paper) | ISBN 9781421428727
(electronic) | ISBN 1421428725 (electronic)
Subjects: | MESH: Obesity—history | History, 20th Century | United States
Classification: LCC RC628 | NLM WD 210 | DDC 362.1963/9800973—dc23
LC record available at https://lccn.loc.gov/2018033818

A catalog record for this book is available from the British Library.

*Special discounts are available for bulk purchases of this book. For more
information, please contact Special Sales at 410-516-6936 or specialsales@
press.jhu.edu.*

Johns Hopkins University Press uses environmentally friendly book
materials, including recycled text paper that is composed of at least 30
percent post-consumer waste, whenever possible.

Contents

Acknowledgments

This book could not have been written without the time and patience of quite a number of public health experts, including Lisa Bero, Adrian Carter, Tim Gill, Wayne Hall, Bob Kaplan, Lynda Powell, and all my instructors in the MPH program at the University of Sydney School of Public Health. Special thanks to Paul Griffiths at the Charles Perkins Centre, who kindly hosted me as a visiting scholar at that hotbed of health policy work.

It equally could not have been written without the patient help of many archivists, including those at the Center for the History of Medicine at Harvard's Countway Medical Library, the Dwight D. Eisenhower Presidential Library, the Harry S. Truman Presidential Library, the History of Medicine Division of the US National Library of Medicine, the John P. McGovern Historical Research Center of the Houston Academy of Medicine–Texas Medical Center Library, the National Archives at College Park, the Rockefeller Archive Center, the University of California at Los Angeles, and the Woodson Research Center of Rice University's Fondren Library. For generously helping me access other important primary sources I must also thank Mary Hilperthauser of the History Office of the Centers for Disease Control and Prevention, Henry Blackburn of the University of Minnesota, and Paul Sorlie, the keeper of the National Heart, Lung, and Blood Institute's historical memory.

I am deeply indebted to many other researchers in the history of related public health fields, and in the history and philosophy of science more generally, for sharing ideas and information with me in the course of this project. These include Warwick Anderson, Henry Blackburn, Dan Bouk, David Courtwright, Cristin Kearns, Howard Kushner, Michael Lempert, Gerald Oppenheimer, Jessica Parr, Scott Podolsky, Hans Pols, and—again and especially—Paul Griffiths. I have benefited from feedback after sharing my work at many conferences and seminars, most memorably at the University of Toronto and at the Stanford Center for Advanced Studies in Behavioral Sciences, where I was privileged to enjoy a residential fellowship while on sabbatical to begin the writing of this book in 2015.

I am extremely grateful to the Australian Research Council, which supported the bulk of the research presented here with Discovery Project DP140101629, and for a Countway Library Fellowship in History of Medicine from Harvard and the Boston Medical Library at an early stage in the research.

I would like to express my gratitude to those who helped in the writing process to make this a better book, although responsibility for any errors of course remains with me: Jess Parr for her work as a research assistant, Audra Wolfe of the Outside Reader for editorial assistance, anonymous reviewers for their comments, and Robin W. Coleman at Johns Hopkins University Press for his unwavering interest and support.

Finally, I thank my wonderful family—Jackie, Amelie, and Lucie—for encouraging me and giving me space to write.

Fat in the Fifties

CHAPTER 1

Fat and the Public's Health before the Second World War

Anyone who spends much time reading, watching, or listening to health news has encountered a certain type of story. Researchers identify a disease or condition as a leading cause of premature death. Scientists explain its physical causes, and public health authorities advise that adopting some behaviors—and abandoning others—will reduce the risks of contracting (or dying of) this disease because of these causes. If we follow all the advice, we might not only live longer but become "healthier" indefinitely. This kind of thinking about health and disease permeates our contemporary experience and self-understanding. Sociologists have given the phenomenon various names, including the "biomedicalization" of "biopolitics" and the emergence of a "risk society."[1]

From a long historical perspective, this is a profoundly new state of affairs. Prior to the Second World War, national authorities routinely monitored their populations' births and deaths, but not their illnesses or the characteristics and activities of the people most likely to suffer them. Likewise, while laboratory and clinical research certainly existed prior to the war, it developed into the massive, government-funded, self-reinforcing biomedical enterprise of today in the postwar years. Only then did the discipline of public health turn the greatest part of its efforts to shaping an individual's "lifestyle" so as to reduce exposure to the causes of diseases, as interpreted by the new epidemiological and laboratory sciences. In contrast, during the first half of the twentieth century, public health efforts focused on removing hazards (especially infectious agents) from the environment. Biological and clinical research operated largely separately from one another, and mostly were funded by private foundations. And although life expectancies had already grown during this time period, so that the noncommunicable, chronic diseases that generally strike later in life began to predominate, scientists, doctors, and public health authorities continued to concentrate primarily on the communicable diseases that had until recently kept life short by killing the very young and the old at appalling rates.[2]

This book explores these postwar shifts in epidemiology, experimental biomedicine, and public health through the lens of obesity in the United States. Obesity is presently, of course, the topic of one of those stories about the risk of deadly disease and how, through behavioral change, to reduce that risk based on science. But the current obesity epidemic is not the first time that US authorities have warned Americans that their collective excess weight constitutes a major threat. Obesity first emerged as a public health crisis in the early 1950s, only to disappear mysteriously in the late 1960s and early 1970s. The rise and fall of this epidemic cannot be explained biologically: waistlines expanded throughout the twentieth century, and in the twenty-first century Americans are not growing thinner. In this book, I explore the history of the mostly forgotten first obesity epidemic as a politically meaningful and culturally resonant problem. When public health priorities and cultural attitudes shifted in the late 1960s, obesity lost its power to compel action. This story thus reinforces many others in the history of medicine that show that diseases are not fixed, but depend on the economics, politics, healing practices, and ideas of health in the cultures where they appear.

Obesity burst into the public consciousness in the years immediately following the Second World War. Around 1950, the US Public Health Service (PHS) issued a brochure on "the greatest problem in preventive medicine in the USA": obesity. The life insurance industry, working in collaboration with the PHS and the American Medical Association (AMA), launched a national drive, proclaiming "Overweight: America's No. 1 Health Problem." And no wonder, given that insurance company data and some local health surveys suggested that more than a quarter of the American population was significantly overweight or obese. By the typical measure of the day, anyone 10 percent above the "ideal weight" for a given height fell into the category of overweight—the ideal weight being that which the insurance industry found to predict maximum longevity. Those 20 percent overweight were classified as obese. The danger of excess weight was grave, because it was the leading predictor of heart disease, the nation's top killer.

The early postwar period was a unique moment for the nation's health in many ways. In the first two decades of the twentieth century the noncontagious chronic diseases, chief among them heart disease and cancer, had surpassed infectious diseases as the leading causes of death. The rising tide of cancer was recognized by the establishment of the National Cancer Institute in 1937, and the even greater importance of heart disease to the nation's health was recognized by the National Heart

Institute's founding in 1948, a move marking the dramatic expansion of the Na-tional Institutes of Health (NIH). By 1960 the NIH budget had grown to eight times its 1950 level, and the research conducted at or funded by the NIH had won the United States standing as the world's biomedical research superpower. But the drive for research into the dominant causes of heart disease did not start with the govern-ment; rather, it came from the insurance industry, which had the most extensive epidemiological data in the country. Throughout the early postwar period, public health authorities and the medical establishment, led by the AMA, remained locked in a fierce struggle about the state's role in providing health care—specifically, whether the United States would join much of the developed world in supplying its citizens with near-universal health insurance (to be administered by the PHS or its parent agency). Nevertheless, even these warring factions could agree that obesity was a health crisis requiring a major policy initiative. Meanwhile, the new Cold War and the fear of atomic annihilation heightened anxieties about national fitness.

The idea of a deadly obesity epidemic barely lasted a decade. By the end of the 1960s the prevalence of true obesity was being officially downgraded, as was obe-sity's status as a cause of heart disease—for epidemiologists, it was a secondary cause at best or perhaps just a side effect of too much dietary fat, the real cause. This downgrading cannot be attributed to a blanket disinvestment in health: other federal initiatives, including subsidies for hospital construction and the perpetual expansion of the NIH research enterprise, continued (although there was a 1970s plateau). Nor can the virtual disappearance of the obesity epidemic be explained through research findings: public health authorities lost interest in obesity even before strong scientific evidence, now itself undergoing revision, emerged to cast serious doubts on the link between obesity and heart disease. The idea that par-ticular fats in the diet caused coronary heart disease—the diet-heart theory—had taken its place in the limelight.

Given the reemergence of obesity as a public health crisis around 2000, the story of the rise and fall of the first obesity epidemic is of obvious contemporary interest. Why did the alarm bells fade if Americans were growing no thinner and still seemed to be dying from heart disease at massive rates? The story is also of interest for understanding the history, politics, and culture of the postwar United States, especially for understanding the history of medicine and public health in that context. The narrative that follows touches on nearly every aspect of American life, from the popularity of self-help groups meeting in church basements in new suburbs to the establishment of a modern state apparatus that (selectively) began to monitor the health problems of the entire country. This is a tale of a country that lavishly funded laboratory research into the causes of health and illness while taking little action to address the health needs of living citizens. Through examining the rise and fall of the obesity epidemic, we can gain an understanding of how the American public health system—ambitious, strong, and second to none at the end of the Second World War—was constrained a decade later to focus mainly on nagging individuals to change their lifestyle choices.

The first obesity epidemic offers insights into several important trends in twentieth-century medical science. In the 1920s and 1930s, obesity was regarded as a glandular condition; by the 1950s, it was seen as a psychiatric condition closely related to alcoholism and drug addiction. How did this shift come to be, and what does it reveal about medicine's attitude toward individual responsibility and health? At the same time, the transfer of the leadership in epidemiological research from the insurance industry to academic researchers and the US public health establishment meant an increasing focus on biological causes of disease, not just predictive correlations. Laboratory research into the processes related to heart disease became linked to epidemiological studies of the general population. And epidemiological researchers' interest in the biological causes of heart disease steered them toward the role of particular dietary fats. But before this new epidemiology distracted researchers away from obesity in the 1960s, so that the heart disease problem became one of dietary choices, the public health community had by default settled on individual weight loss as its chief approach to the nation's leading killer.[3]

New biomedical ideas about obesity and illness found their way into public consciousness in ways that intensified social pressure to maintain slimness, particularly among women (even though the rise in heart disease was seen mainly as a male problem). Cast as a disease of the will and emotions—the soul—by the Freudian psychiatry of the early postwar era, obesity became a highly visible character defect, stigmatizing those considered fat.[4] It was mainly women, already blamed by that same psychiatry for many of society's ills in their roles as faulty mothers, who responded to the new messages of physical health, virtue, beauty, and mental health by pursuing weight loss through self-help (or, better, mutual aid) clubs. Weight-loss groups appeared in a range of forms, including those that reflected the era's infatuation with introspective psychiatry, those that adopted the confessional-spiritual model of Alcoholics Anonymous, and those that appealed to biomedical authority. Since these clubs also met a variety of social needs for their participants, the story of their rise provides a glimpse into the experiences and values of the women who populated the nation's new and sprawling suburbia.

The virtual disappearance of obesity as a public health problem in the 1960s shows that dangers and crises hinge on selective attention and on values. By then, experts had shifted their focus to particular dietary fats as the primary lifestyle contributors to heart disease. The Kennedy and Johnson administrations, meanwhile, shifted the country's public health programming away from questions of the moral fiber and fitness of the middle classes and toward improving access to food, housing, and health care services for the poor. The obesity epidemic ended when a new definition of overweight—body-mass index (BMI)—replaced the prior categorization based on actuarial tables. Whereas the insurance industry had defined obesity as deviation from a height and weight combination that predicted long life, BMI was a measure simply of weight for height, agnostic in itself about health implications. Outside the halls of medicine, the popular stigma surrounding obesity declined sharply in the early 1970s in the midst of broader societal changes that embraced a much wider range of identities and lifestyles than had previously been socially acceptable. Against a backdrop of evidence that suggested that mortality from heart disease was no longer accelerating, in the 1970s public health authorities turned their attention toward cancer. Obesity thus became a neglected problem— until, of course, it resurfaced in the 1990s, when most histories of the problem begin.[5]

I begin my account of the US obesity epidemic in an earlier period, the 1920s and 1930s, a time of great optimism and experimentation in the realm of public health. Health authorities, in alliance with the insurance industry, explored how to approach a new era in which chronic diseases, heart disease chief among them, had become the greatest threat. It was in this context that the obesity alarm was first sounded. I then explore the surprising transformation of obesity from glandular to mental illness, together with the implications for its control. In the middle of the book I describe how a national campaign against obesity was mobilized and the complex ways in which it interacted with a fierce political and policy battle over government's role in health care. After looking at some of that campaign's effects on people considered fat, I turn to the changes—cultural, commercial, political, and scientific—that undermined obesity as a matter of grave concern.

New Deal Public Health and Its Clash with Medicine

Understanding how the United States came to find itself in the midst of an obesity epidemic in 1950 requires a closer look at the changing politics of public health in the twentieth century. In the years immediately following the Second World War, the public health and medical communities were locked in a conflict about the proper role of the state in providing care for its citizens. The contours of that debate reflected not only the new politics of socialized medicine in the face of the Cold War, but also the legacy of President Franklin Delano Roosevelt. A host of New Deal programs had expanded the social safety net in the 1930s and 1940s, including broader provision of public health services. What would be the fate of those programs during a rising wave of anticommunism?

Roosevelt arrived in office in 1933 with a mandate to enlarge the power of the federal government so as to improve the public welfare and to rescue the economy from the depths of the Great Depression. One of his leading successes on the welfare front was the Social Security Act, passed into law in 1935. Best known for providing some income for retired workers, the measure was originally conceived as a more ambitious social insurance plan along European lines, including provisions for near-universal health insurance. Rumors of universal health care sparked such vociferous opposition from the American Medical Association, however, that the Roosevelt administration dropped the medical aspect of Social Security to ease the measure's passage through Congress. The AMA opposed government interference in doctors' work as independent businessmen, as it would for the rest of the twentieth century.[6]

Roosevelt nevertheless remained concerned about the issue, and some members of his administration sought other opportunities to incorporate national health insurance into the New Deal. One result was the appointment of the Interdepartmental Committee to Coordinate Health and Welfare Activities, which created a subcommittee to study the health status and needs of the nation. The study's recommendations, which were presented in July 1938 at an event in Washington, DC, marking the 141st anniversary of the PHS, called for a dramatic expansion of federal funding and services, including new public health, maternal health, and child health services; new hospital facilities; federal assistance for state programs providing health services to those unable to pay; federally funded disability insurance; and, most controversially, "a general program of medical care, paid either through general taxation or social insurance contributions" (as with Social Security). While organized medicine bitterly opposed this last recommendation, organized labor appeared enthusiastic about the prospect of increased federal involvement in the nation's health.[7]

Over the next few years, several bills based on the committee's vision made their way through Congress. The most prominent was an omnibus health bill introduced in early 1939, which was known as the Wagner bill after its sponsor in the Senate, New York Democrat Robert F. Wagner. A New Deal champion, Wagner had previously sponsored the version of the Social Security legislation that eventually became law. The Wagner bill proposed to revise the Social Security Act to encompass more health matters, increase funding for the Public Health Service and the Children's Bureau, and allow (but not require) the states to establish public medical insurance programs funded by the federal government through the PHS. Although the bill died in committee for lack of Roosevelt's unequivocal support, the administration reorganized the executive branch as a step toward realizing its broader social security vision. That year, the Social Security Administration, the Public Health Service, the Food and Drug Administration, and other major agencies with health functions were moved into the new Federal Security Agency (FSA); in 1946, the Children's Bureau would move as well. Thus a new federal administrative apparatus to manage public health, health care, retirement, disability, and other welfare functions had already been created by the time the United States entered the war.[8]

In 1943 Wagner and two colleagues, James E. Murray from Montana and John D. Dingell of Michigan, introduced a new national health insurance bill. The Wagner-Murray-Dingell bill proposed universal federal health insurance, which would be administered by the Public Health Service and its chief, the surgeon general, but implemented through the states. Once again, the AMA mounted a vigorous opposition. Killed in committee, the bill was revised and reintroduced in 1945. The FSA officials who drafted these bills put the PHS at the center of a state-managed national health system. By the time that Harry Truman came to occupy the Oval Office in mid-1945, the Public Health Service—and, by extension, public health generally—had become thoroughly associated with the "socialized medicine" that many American physicians dreaded and despised. This connection would hamper the progress of public health generally in the United States for years to come.[9]

The New Public Health

The field of public health had expansionary visions during the Roosevelt and Truman administrations. When New Deal and Fair Deal officials advocated for universal health care, they were drawing on ideas and plans developed by public health leaders of the 1920s and 1930s. By the end of the First World War, public health could claim triumphant success in controlling major infectious diseases through aggressive efforts to reduce the health hazards of the urban environment. Particularly in New York and other large cities, public health authorities had gained control over sewage, water supplies, garbage, and tenement housing. An improved knowledge of bacteriology allowed health departments to drive down death rates by monitoring and containing the spread of contagious diseases like typhoid, by establishing medical examinations for students and placing nurses in schools, by distributing safe milk to mothers and inspecting the safety of commercial milk, and even by manufacturing vaccines and antitoxins in direct competition with the then-dubious pharmaceutical industry.[10]

Public health professionals gained ground against chronic diseases as well. Syphilis and tuberculosis are infectious diseases that can take years to cure. Both served as experimental spaces where researchers could apply techniques derived from infectious disease control to the emerging problems of noncommunicable disease management. The techniques that public health departments developed to address these problems included large-scale screening drives that provided free examinations to entire communities at once, the establishment of public sanatoriums and clinics to which indigent patients could be referred for treatment, sending public health nurses to follow up on discovered cases, and compulsory reporting requirements for all people diagnosed with syphilis and, in some states, tuberculosis.[11] This reporting enabled health departments to ensure that all cases on their registers received treatment and to trace their contacts to check for disease transmission.

To C.-E. Winslow, a progressive leader of early twentieth-century American public health and head of an influential department at Yale, the campaigns for sanitation and infection control were all but won. In 1920, it seemed obvious to him that the next step was to erase the "artificial boundary line between public health and private medicine" so that preventive and therapeutic health care could be co-ordinated and delivered in a fashion that was maximally efficient for society. One of his mentors, Hermann Biggs of the New York City public health department, had formulated a plan to do just that. Biggs proposed that municipal governments establish health care centers, funded by the state but administered by local health departments, where all citizens could obtain a full range of preventive and therapeutic services from doctors and nurses employed by the city. Fees would be affordable and could be waived for those unable to pay. Resistance from the medical profession blocked this proposal from coming into law in New York state. Nevertheless, Biggs's idea to organize clinical practice and make it responsive to public health was widely influential between the wars. Winslow and other progressives in his circle advanced many health reform proposals based on this general model, and it even achieved something close to an endorsement from US Surgeon General Hugh Cumming in the mid-1920s.[12]

Some interwar reformers in public health went further than this, arguing that clinical medicine should be fully subordinate to public health. Better yet, both medicine and public health should be amalgamated into a larger enterprise often called "social medicine." The idea was implemented in the new Soviet Union during the 1920s in a program to uncover and correct the causes of health disparities through welfare actions, preventive services, and clinical care—ultimately, social engineering to improve health. Although the program did not last long in the Soviet Union, a number of Western medical reformers observed the experiment and reported what they found. The model became particularly influential in England, where a camp of public health reformers established social medicine as a discipline in the universities. The vision of social medicine played an important role in the establishment of several postwar institutions, including the British National Health Service and the international World Health Organization. In the United States, the Milbank Fund, a foundation established in 1905, incorporated social medicine into its mission of improving health through social reform.[13]

Even among those public health authorities whose vision fell short of sweeping reforms along social medicine lines, there emerged a broad consensus that social conditions, combined with personal behavior, determined health in the domain of chronic diseases. Already by the 1920s, Winslow had perceived that chronic disease demanded that public health authorities shift their attention, at least partially, from the environment to individual behavior: "the primary interest of the health officer," he said, must now go to "the detection of non-contagious physical defects and the hygienic guidance of the individual living machine." And if public health were to focus on the conditions taking the greatest toll, so as to achieve the maximum health benefit for the minimum cost—as Winslow thought it should—it would have to find ways to attack heart disease, the king of chronic illnesses.[14] But accomplishing this task would require public health authorities to know much more than they currently did about the distribution and causes of heart disease, along with other chronic illnesses. The task demanded a new epidemiology.

Mortality Rates and the New Epidemiology

During the period between the wars and in the immediate postwar period, public health and medicine knew more about what was killing people than about what conditions accounted for sickness, especially chronic or prolonged illness. The United States had established a national system for recording mortality data from standardized death certificates in the first decade of the twentieth century, but it took until 1933 for this practice to reach all corners of the nation. The reporting system was, moreover, prone to uncertainty, both from changes in disease classification and from variations over time and space in the thinking of the physicians recording the main cause of death on the certificates. The death certificate data had the virtue of reflecting essentially the whole population, but had the defect of being much more informative about people's overall health as reflected in their lifespans than about whose health was impaired by what conditions and at what times in their lives. To explore health and sickness among the living, during the 1920s and 1930s epidemiologists developed methods for surveying morbidity.

Using the older death certificate data, government (and other) statisticians showed a gratifying decline in mortality rates in the 1920s. Life expectancy at birth (a conveniently calculable measure of typical lifespan) had, since the turn of the twentieth century, increased by a decade to around fifty-five. Statisticians attributed the steadily declining death rate to the retreat of infectious diseases, especially those that most strongly affected early childhood, including diphtheria and dysentery.[15] It appeared that public health measures had cleaned up urban environments enough to make them nearly as healthful as the countryside, which housed an ever-diminishing proportion of the population as the nation industrialized. (This was the situation for white people—the mortality rate of the country's African American population actually increased in the early twentieth century, most likely because of segregated housing conditions that produced extreme crowding in cities.)[16] The health of industrial workers also was showing great improvement. According to one study by statistician Louis Dublin, using data from the Metropolitan Life Insurance Company of New York, during the decade between 1912 and 1923 the life expectancy of a white, twenty-year-old working man increased by five years.[17] All told, the picture of American health emerging from mortality statistics appeared rosy.

Louis Dublin is a character worth getting to know better, and not only because he emerges time and again in this book as a voice pointing to obesity as a factor undermining health in America. Dublin's career illustrates the key role that the insurance industry played in both epidemiology and public health in the early twentieth century. Immigrating to New York from Lithuania as a child in 1886, Dublin worked his way through City College of New York and then moved on to Columbia, where he earned a PhD in biostatistics in 1904. In 1908 he left a job teaching at City College for a position under the medical director of Mutual Life Insurance. Obesity was already under suspicion as a risk and as a reason for higher life insurance premiums, and Dublin's new employer wanted to determine more precisely how much extra to charge overweight customers because of their elevated mortality rate. Based on a new study analyzing hundreds of thousands of previous policyholders, Dublin helped compile one of the first tables of normal (i.e., average) weights that included men and women of every height and age. Thus began a career-long fascination with the health penalties of obesity.[18]

In 1909, Dublin moved to the new Welfare Division of Metropolitan Life Insurance. This unique undertaking aspired to increase profits by improving the health of MetLife's "industrial" policyholders: working-class people with small policies, whose premiums were collected by the door-to-door salesmen who sold the policies. The Welfare Division's programs blended public health and social work by, for instance, sending free visiting nurses to these underserved customers. Metropolitan soon became the largest life insurer in the country, and Dublin not only helped his firm do well by doing good, but also served science by studying the firm's data on the lives and deaths of millions of policyholders—a data set far better than what was then available to public health professionals in both quantity and richness. Dublin remained at Metropolitan for forty-three years, becoming head statistician and later a vice president. By the time he retired, he was a gray eminence of the public health community, a leading health policy reformer, and a public intellectual known for articles and speeches on such topics as "can we extend the lifespan?" and books like *The Facts of Life*—all reflecting his pioneering research into the health conditions that shortened lives and reduced productivity (which were not necessarily the same).[19]

The statistical work produced by Dublin and others made clear that life-extending advances in public health, coupled with a declining birth rate, had shifted the main causes of death in the United States. The significance of this change in the causes of death was not appreciated as quickly as the decline in the overall death rate. When people survive to an older age, they tend to succumb to noninfectious illnesses, many of which are progressive conditions that only become symptomatic in later years. Stroke, cancer, and, most of all, heart disease leaped to the forefront as causes of death.[20] By 1920 heart disease had taken the lead as the top cause of death; by the end of the decade, based mainly on evidence developed by Dublin and other insurance industry statisticians, health policy analysts came to believe that heart disease was also catching up with tuberculosis in terms of its total financial burden on the nation (despite the fact that heart disease tended to kill its victims later in their wage-earning years). Imposing double the economic burden of cancer, which would soon become the second greatest cause of death, heart disease had unquestionably become Public Health Enemy Number 1 by 1930.[21]

The insurance industry had an additional set of mortality statistics beyond death certificates, which was not available to public health authorities. Since the late nineteenth century, most insurance companies had required applicants to

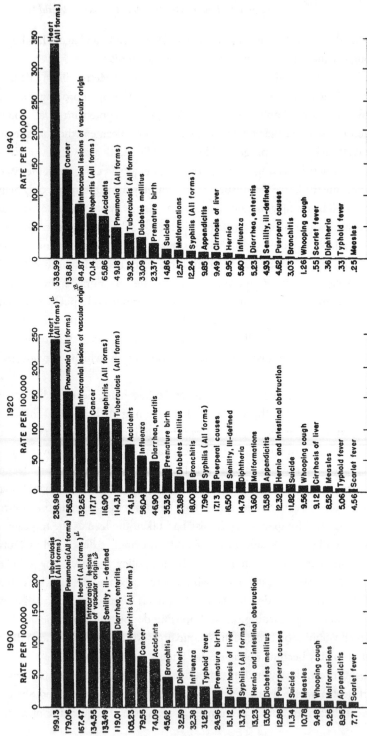

FIGURE 2.—Comparative rank of age-adjusted rates for major causes of death, in the death registration States of 1900, for 1900, 1920, and 1940. Rates are adjusted to the age distribution of the total population, enumerated, 1940.

[1] Excludes diseases of coronary arteries.　　[2] Includes all embolism and thrombosis, except puerperal.

complete a standard medical examination before enrollment. They used the results of the exam to set premiums and reject particularly bad risks. But the practice also provided insurance companies with prospective data that they could later compare against an enrollee's cause of death—and perhaps improve future risk assessment.[22]

At the turn of the twentieth century, insurance companies began pooling such data, using them to conduct increasingly sophisticated statistical analyses in search of early predictors of poor longevity. In the landmark Medico-Actuarial Mortality Investigation (MAMI), a consortium of firms pooled data from more than 440,000 policies (representing an equal number of men and women) issued from 1885 through 1900 and observed to the policy anniversaries in 1909. This was the data set young Dublin drew on when he developed his first height-weight tables. MAMI was followed by the similarly designed and executed Medical Impairment study, which included data on 667,000 men who were issued policies from 1909 through 1927 and were followed to their policy anniversaries in 1928. Both of these studies mainly looked at overall mortality rates associated with occupations or obvious "impairments," only rarely attempting to identify predictors of particular causes of death (quite prudently, given the variability in how doctors completed death certificates). The findings indicated a clear association between overweight and excess mortality. In the 1929 Medical Impairment study, men 25 percent or more above average weight for their height suffered 30–40 percent higher mortality rates, depending on their age. In a study led by Dublin ten years later, Metropolitan found similar results for women, although the mortality penalties of excess weight were not quite as severe as for men. Based on the interwar studies, the insurance firms updated their height-weight tables to reflect greater mortality penalties for overweight and smaller mortality penalties for underweight. Tuberculosis, which slowly made people thin before killing them, was in retreat.[23]

In 1930, Louis Dublin used this type of information as the basis for a groundbreaking actuarial study that specifically correlated overweight with heart disease. Noting that death certificate recording had improved greatly since the MAMI study

Opposite, The leading causes of death between 1900 and 1940 in the United States (age structure normalized to 1940), showing the dramatic decline of infectious diseases and the transition to dominance of heart disease, stroke, and cancer. *Note*: In 1900 and 1920, the heart disease rate excluded coronary heart disease, a condition much more commonly entered on death certificates in later years. Reprinted from I. M. Moriyama and Mary Gover, "Statistical Studies of Heart Diseases: I. Heart Diseases and Allied Causes of Death in Relation to Age Changes in the Population," *Public Health Reports* 63, no. 17 (1948): 537–545.

Standardized Death Rates per 100,000 *for Specified Causes of Death—All Ages Combined—By Weight Classes*

CAUSES OF DEATH	DEATHRATE PER 100,000		
	Under-weights	Normals	Overweights
All causes	848	844	1,111
Circulatory diseases			
Organic diseases of heart	65	80	121
Angina pectoris	14	16	35
Diseases of the arteries	17	23	38
Acute endocarditis and pericarditis	6	8	13
Nephritis, acute and chronic	63	82	141
Cerebral hemorrhage and apoplexy	49	70	110
Paralysis	12	14	17
Cancer	62	61	68
Diabetes	9	14	36
Tuberculosis, all forms	126	64	30
Pulmonary tuberculosis	115	57	26
Respiratory diseases			
Pneumonia, lobar and unspecified	70	63	59
Broncho-pneumonia	5	6	7
Influenza	20	20	28
Diseases of the digestive system			
Appendicitis	15	17	20
Cirrhosis of the liver	9	9	15
Typhoid fever	28	29	39
General paralysis of insane	12	11	14
External causes			
Accidents	55	60	67
Suicides	27	24	31

By 1930 the life insurance industry found that the elevated risks of overweight and obesity had outstripped the risks of underweight and were especially apparent in excess heart disease, stroke, kidney disease, and diabetes. Reprinted from table 5 in "The Influence of Weight on Certain Causes of Death" by L. Dublin, in *Human Biology: The International Journal of Population Genetics and Anthropology* 2, no. 2. Copyright © 1930 Wayne State University Press, with the permission of Wayne State University Press.

(whose analyses of cause of death were regarded as questionable), Dublin looked at particular causes of death among 192,000 men insured between 1887 and 1908 and followed to 1921 or policy termination. The sample was especially uniform and, in today's terms, free of confounding variables: all subjects were male, white, from the Midwest region, and not engaged in industrial labor or other dangerous occupations. Dublin confirmed earlier findings that overweight men suffered higher overall mortality, and he showed that this excess mortality increased smoothly with the degree of overweight, as one would expect with exposure to any harmful condition.[24] The effects were more pronounced in men over forty-five. More unexpected was Dublin's finding that the excess mortality from overweight could be attributed to only a handful of causes, chief among them heart diseases. For cardiovascular (heart and artery) diseases combined, for stroke, and also for diabetes, even men just 5 percent to 14 percent above average weight for their heights suffered an extra mortality penalty of around 50 percent. Excess mortality from kidney disease was nearly as high—understandably, given that the chief causes of kidney disease are diabetes and heart disease. And of course the death toll from all these conditions was even worse for those 15 percent or more overweight.[25]

A Glimpse into Chronic Illness

But what of the health of the living? For most of the period covered in this book, mortality statistics remained the main driver of health policy in the United States. Nevertheless, new methods to assess and respond to morbidity emerged during this time. In 1915, Metropolitan Life Insurance began a major two-year study on the prevalence of various illnesses among living people. The Metropolitan investigators, led by Dublin, surveyed half a million members of policyholding families about their health condition on a particular day. Shortly afterward in the course of studies on pellagra, a debilitating nutritional deficiency rampant among southern cotton workers, the Public Health Service adopted a similar form of cross-sectional health survey. Both of these studies attempted to measure the contribution of different illnesses to absenteeism at work. The fact that poverty correlated strongly with absenteeism suggested that poverty itself was a cause of ill health.[26]

Reflecting the new interest of Progressive Era public health in reducing the general burden of disease on society, between 1921 and 1924 the PHS conducted the first comprehensive American survey of morbidity. For its sample, PHS chose the "typical" (more than 90 percent native-born white) and conveniently located town of Hagerstown, Maryland. PHS representatives fanned out to 1,800 households, representing about a quarter of the town's population, assessing the characteristics of residents such as "color, sex and age"; their "general economic status, sanitary condition, method of excreta disposal"; and water and milk sources. Then they conducted return visits every six to eight weeks over the course of twenty-eight months, asking residents what periods of sickness they could recall since the preceding

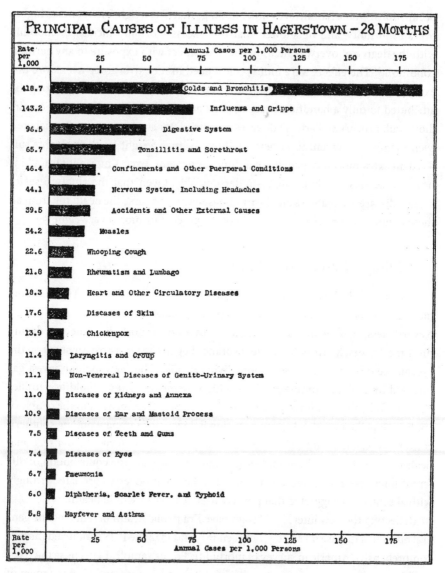

PRINCIPAL CAUSES OF ILLNESS IN HAGERSTOWN.—28 MONTHS

Rate per 1,000	Annual Cases per 1,000 Persons
418.7	Colds and Bronchitis
143.2	Influenza and Grippe
96.5	Digestive System
65.7	Tonsillitis and Sorethroat
46.4	Confinements and Other Puerperal Conditions
44.1	Nervous System, Including Headaches
39.5	Accidents and Other External Causes
34.2	Measles
22.6	Whooping Cough
21.8	Rheumatism and Lumbago
18.3	Heart and Other Circulatory Diseases
17.6	Diseases of Skin
13.9	Chickenpox
11.4	Laryngitis and Croup
11.1	Non-Venereal Diseases of Genito-Urinary System
11.0	Diseases of Kidneys and Annexa
10.9	Diseases of Ear and Mastoid Process
7.5	Diseases of Teeth and Gums
7.4	Diseases of Eyes
6.7	Pneumonia
6.0	Diphtheria, Scarlet Fever, and Typhoid
5.8	Hayfever and Asthma

Morbidity is represented by the frequency of disability episodes as recalled by surveyed people; note the dominance of transitory respiratory infections. Reprinted from E. Sydenstricker, "A Study of Illness in a General Population Group: Hagerstown Morbidity Studies No. I: The Method of Study and General Results," *Public Health Reports* 41, no. 39 (1926): 2069–2088.

interval. When residents reported that they had had contact with a physician, the researchers followed up for an independent account of the illness. The researchers also collected data from school absences, notifiable disease reports, and clinic visits. Their goal was to learn the extent to which particular health conditions were causing absences from work and other significant disability.

The number of illness episodes recorded was about equal to the number of "person-years" exposed; that is, on average, everyone in the town reported one disabling period of sickness per year. Unsurprisingly, given the long intervals between survey visits (during which minor ailments might be forgotten), the vast majority (80 percent) of the illnesses recalled and recorded were significant enough to have caused disability for three or more days, 60 percent of them for more than a week. Forty percent were severe enough to cause confinement to bed. But the Hagerstown study was designed to assess not the gravity of various illnesses or even their prevalence, but their rate of *incidence* as causes of distinct episodes of disability. By this measure, as causes of acute but mostly transitory disability episodes, respiratory infections (colds, flu, grippe, bronchitis) were by far the most frequent reason that Americans missed school, work, or other duties. The researchers noted the curious fact that respiratory infections caused 61 percent of illness episodes, but only 20 percent of deaths in Hagerstown during the period. Circulatory and kidney diseases, in contrast, caused 35 percent of deaths but less than 3 percent of illness episodes. These findings clearly signified "the unsuitability of mortality statistics as any indication of the causes of morbidity."[27]

One of the leaders of the Hagerstown study was Edgar Sydenstricker, an eminent epidemiologist who had been involved in the PHS's study of pellagra and would later serve on the New Deal health reform committee mentioned above. In 1928, Sydenstricker left the government's employ to become more directly involved in health policy as the scientific director of the Milbank Fund. Sydenstricker used his position at Milbank to organize another morbidity study in the form of a collaboration between PHS and several private foundations. This study, known as the Committee on the Costs of Medical Care (CCMC), surveyed 9,000 families in eighteen states from 1928 to 1931.[28] The CCMC employed a design similar to that of the Hagerstown study, but with special attention to medical services and expenses. The CCMC study's findings also resembled those of Hagerstown, except that respiratory infections did not quite outweigh all other causes of illness combined. But by the authors' own admission the survey was, like Hagerstown, poorly suited to capture illness from chronic disease, since it neglected lower-grade illnesses in favor of well-marked episodes of especially bad health.[29]

The main importance of the CCMC study, however, was not in the findings themselves, but in how the authors proposed to address them. The membership of the CCMC included both public health reformers and those aligned with the mainstream medical profession. After issuing many reports, the committee issued two sets of recommendations, which reflected the split between the two professional groups. The public health reformers, who were the majority of the CCMC's authors, recommended that health insurance be made universally available. They additionally recommended "organized" medical practice, a vague category of the time that included private health insurance plans but also might include state-managed care. The medical faction rejected the idea of organized or group practice, insisting that medicine should remain an individual, strictly fee-for-service enterprise. According to Louis Dublin, who participated in the study as a planner, a researcher, and an executive board member, the minority report came as a complete surprise to the CCMC's leadership. As he recalled, the minority report, engineered and written by the American Medical Association and announced at the last minute, signified medicine's turn away from science and public service and toward petty business interests—it was the moment when medicine "won a signal victory but lost its soul." The medical profession was becoming an enemy of any collective effort to improve the nation's health, with profound impact on the future of obesity control and on public health more generally.[30]

Undeterred by the AMA's resistance, Sydenstricker brought his interest in morbidity surveys to the Roosevelt administration. Working as a consultant to the PHS (and a mentor to the PHS officers involved), Sydenstricker led the drive for a massive National Health Survey designed to make the case for national health insurance. As historian George Weisz has shown, Sydenstricker and his collaborators at the PHS were certain that a careful study of morbidity (as opposed to mortality) would substantiate the theory that poverty was making people sick. Since people living in poverty could not afford medical care, they suffered worse health outcomes when they got sick, which meant that they missed work for longer periods of time— thereby reinforcing the cycle. When Sydenstricker first proposed the National Health Survey early in the New Deal, there was little existing evidence for an association between poverty and illness (findings from Hagerstown supporting it had not yet been published, and mortality statistics suggested that the Depression had, if anything, improved longevity).[31] The project's advocates nevertheless hoped that the sheer scale of poverty emerging from the Great Depression would yield evidence justifying an expansion of public health and publicly funded health services.[32]

It certainly highlighted the new public health's ambitions to address the social conditions impairing society's health.

In many ways the National Health Survey followed the design of the Hagerstown and CCMC surveys, but its scale and explicit interest in addressing poverty produced different results. Conducted in 1935 and 1936 with unprecedented federal funding from the Works Progress Administration, the National Health Survey was two orders of magnitude larger than the prior studies, ultimately visiting 700,000 urban families in eighteen states and 37,000 rural families in three states. Altogether, the survey reported on the health of 2.8 million participants. The methodology differed in several key ways from the prior studies as well. Because of the scale of the survey, the 6,000 "enumerators" who called on the sampled families made only a single visit; they relied on information retrieved from 400,000 physician reports to confirm participants' accounts of serious illness. Whereas surveyors in Hagerstown recorded any illness significant to the participants, the National Health Survey's enumerators asked about episodes of illness disabling enough to have caused hospitalization or absence from work, school, or other normal duties for seven days in the previous year. This line of questioning naturally drew attention to more severe illnesses than prior surveys had. But perhaps the most important difference was that enumerators also made note of certain chronic illnesses even if they had not caused disability as strictly defined. These conditions included asthma, cancer, nephritis or kidney disease, rheumatism or arthritis, tuberculosis, and heart disease—all of which had been overshadowed in the previous morbidity surveys.[33]

With its stress on recording seriously disabling illnesses as well as prespecified chronic diseases, the National Health Survey yielded a very different picture of American health than had previous health surveys. Even with a new, more stringent definition of illness, respiratory complaints remained the most frequent cause of illness episodes lasting at least seven days. However, measured by "volume" or average days of disability per year in the general population (that is, among the sickness episodes causing seven days or more of disability), heart disease ranked at the top, followed by mental disease, and then orthopedic impairment. Nonspecific acute respiratory complaints now came in fourth rather than first place. Among the causes of disability lasting for an entire year or more, heart disease again came first and mental illness was a close second; together with the distant third, arthritis, these long-term conditions accounted for more than half of the illnesses creating long-term disability. The survey also showed what Sydenstricker had hoped it would: the unemployed and those experiencing poverty disproportionately suffered

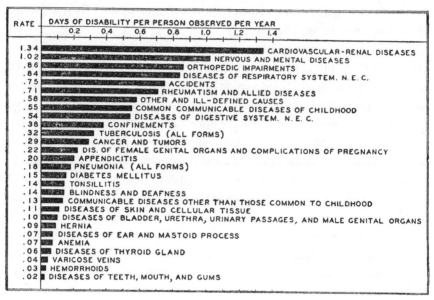

FIGURE 1.—Disability rate by diagnosis for illnesses disabling for one week or longer.

Morbidity is represented by the number of days of disability for episodes lasting longer than seven days as recalled by participants in the National Health Survey. Note how this measure brought heart disease to the fore (cf. figs. 1.1 and 1.3). Reprinted from Rollo Britten, Selwyn Collins, and James Fitzgerald, "The National Health Survey: Some General Findings as to Disease, Accidents, and Impairments in Urban Areas," *Public Health Reports* 55, no. 11 (1940): 444–470.

the burden of disease, much of it of the chronic variety. Contrary to expectation, however, the greatest number of people suffering from serious chronic disease were middle-aged, not elderly.[34]

Several other morbidity studies conducted in the next decade confirmed this rough picture. In 1943, for example, the PHS conducted a follow-up study in Hagerstown that managed to recontact (or find death certificates for) an astonishing 1,628 of the 1,822 families originally surveyed. Its findings confirmed not only that chronic disease was more common among poorer families but that illness evidently *caused* poverty. Of the families reporting chronic disease in 1923 or 1943, around 9 percent had suffered a decline in socioeconomic status by 1943; no similar economic decline was apparent for families that did not report chronic disease at either time. While heart disease lagged behind arthritis and neuritis in prevalence, the survey found heart disease to be the most lethal of these conditions.[35]

Collectively, new epidemiological methods, combined with New Deal efforts to expand the federal government's health programs, revealed chronic illnesses and especially heart disease to be major public health problems. Even conservative analysts leery of the new morbidity data's association with social justice, like the AMA's Morris Fishbein, had to admit that heart disease posed a major threat to Americans' health and economic productivity. The growing expert interest in heart disease set the stage for a major national campaign to understand, prevent, and cure this category of disease once the Second World War finished in 1945. This campaign would move obesity, a prime suspect thanks to the insurance industry's epidemiology, into a harsh spotlight.

Although ample justification was available both in the robust insurance statistics around overweight adults and heart disease and in the population mortality and morbidity profile of heart disease, the years prior to the Second World War saw little agitation about obesity among public health professionals. One may speculate that in the context of the Great Depression and the Roosevelt administration's socioeconomic justice agenda, the problems of poverty and health care access were more interesting and opportune for public health's leaders, and any attention to a seeming disease of affluence was inexpedient. Still, to Dublin, second to none in his mastery of heart disease statistics, 1941 offered a dire picture compared to the long-term successes of public health: while public health authorities might make further gains against syphilitic and rheumatic heart disease by controlling the infectious agents that caused them, the bulk of heart disease mortality and morbidity now came from hypertensive and atherosclerotic (hardened artery) heart disease, and these seemed to derive from natural aging processes. Indeed, by the late 1930s atherosclerotic heart disease (today usually called coronary heart disease, or CHD) had become the leading specific cause of heart disease death, and it was rising. While Dublin and like-minded colleagues held that better "living habits" might retard "degenerative" processes of aging, like the atherosclerosis associated with CHD, the aging of the population inexorably foretold a growing burden of chronic disease so great it could only be managed by state-funded clinical and nursing services. To those who wanted to see an expanded role of government in health, like Sydenstricker, this was a powerful argument in favor of public health's involvement in clinical care, perhaps in a national fleet of chronic disease hospitals.[36]

Yet other, more optimistic voices believed that heart disease might be conquered through medical research. During the interwar period, powerful voluntary health agencies sprang up to advocate on behalf of certain diseases, collecting money for victims and for research to conquer their foes. While heart disease did not yet have a public voice comparable to those that championed the fight against tuberculosis, cancer, or polio, cardiologists watched these parallel efforts with interest. A government report put the 1943 annual fundraising receipts of the National Tuberculosis Association (now the American Lung Association) at $668,000 and those of the American Cancer Society at about $150,000. The recently created National Foundation for Infantile Paralysis brought in a whopping $2,793,000—more than five times the operating budget of the National Cancer Institute that same year—thanks to its phenomenally successful March of Dimes campaign against polio. By comparison, the cardiologists and public health doctors serving as heart disease's spokesmen, organized as the American Heart Association (AHA), had a mere $31,000 to spend. This soon would change.[37]

The AHA's leaders took particular note of the American Cancer Society's success in attracting federal research dollars. Cancer had marched right behind heart disease to the top of the list of leading causes of death as chronic illness overtook infectious disease at the beginning of the century. Between the wars, the American Society for the Control of Cancer, as the American Cancer Society was called until 1944, enjoyed effective leadership in the form of entrepreneurial scientists like Clarence "C. C." Little (then a well-known geneticist, now remembered for inappropriately close ties to the tobacco industry); support from concerned citizens in the advertising and publishing industries; and the dedication of philanthropists and women's clubs, which ran large drives for small donations. The prominent, concerned citizens leading the Cancer Society became a new species of health lobbyist with an unprecedented capacity for mobilizing media as well as money and voters. In 1937 they achieved a stunning political victory when Congress authorized the establishment of the National Cancer Institute, which would be housed in Bethesda, Maryland. The NCI's annual budget of $700,000 (plus an additional $750,000 for construction) represented a new kind of federal investment in medical research. This independent research institute and hospital was combined with the existing national Hygienic Laboratory and became the National Institutes of Health.[38]

Following the cancer advocates' playbook, advocates for heart disease would eventually win their own institute. First, however, they needed to raise the condition's public profile. Only with the Depression and the urgency of war issues, like syphilis and rheumatic disease among servicemen, behind it would the nation be prepared to care more about the ills of affluence and middle age.

CHAPTER 2

Obesity Becomes a Mental Disorder

Imagine two doctors' appointments two decades apart. In each, a forty-five-year-old woman asks her doctor for help losing weight. The first one, in 1928, is told that she's probably having trouble "reducing"—to use the language of the time—because of a glandular condition. She is referred to an endocrinologist and ends up taking hormones to adjust her "slow" metabolism. The second, in 1948, is advised to see a psychiatrist to learn to keep her impulses and emotions under control.

The recognition in the 1930s of heart disease as a major killer linked to obesity coincided with a profound shift in the way fatness and its drivers were understood, both in medicine and in popular culture. Since the turn of the twentieth century, fatness had fallen under the authority of one of the most fashionable and prestigious medical domains of the day, endocrinology. Overweight people were perhaps a source of popular mirth or subjected to scorn, but they were not necessarily responsible for their fate. By the postwar period, however, medical authorities had all but abandoned endocrinological explanations in favor of psychiatric models. To these doctors and researchers, it seemed patently obvious that obesity was caused by overeating, a form of addiction that required explanation in terms of mental disorder or character defect.

Psychiatric theories of obesity fell on fertile ground in the late 1940s for several reasons. Across America, concern about mental health skyrocketed after the war. Health authorities, including US surgeon general Thomas Parran, declared that unrecognized mental illness was rife and responsible for half of the nation's total burden of illness. There was a crisis around overflowing asylums, which were likened to Nazi concentration camps in their squalor and cruelty. As the Cold War developed and the nation turned inward in a search for domestic peace and self-fulfillment, Freudian psychoanalysis along with several other forms of psychological theory penetrated the churches, schools, and popular culture. The Cold War also heightened worries about the mental fitness of Americans for their long struggle with communism, especially concerns that imbalanced or overbearing mothers (so central in Freudian theory) were producing weakness and delinquency in their children. And loosely psychoanalytic, Freud-influenced psychiatry was the flavor of the month in medicine too.[1] And for many doctors and public health professionals concerned about obesity, these psychiatric theories must have been attractive because they opened the notoriously difficult problem of weight loss to practical intervention far more than had the previous endocrinological theory, which typically entailed expensive, ongoing drug treatments from a specialist.

A Glandular Gold Rush

The medical community's embrace of endocrinology in the early twentieth century might have surprised those familiar with the field's dubious origins. In 1889 an aging, eminent French physiologist named Charles-Édouard Brown-Séquard announced that injecting himself with extracts of animal testicles had restored his virility and vigor. Entrepreneurial doctors soon established "organotherapy" practices to capitalize on this latest fountain of youth, triggering a short-lived craze in upper-class circles. The study of the ductless glands—those that function by secreting substances into the bloodstream or tissue fluids—was almost stifled by the charlatanism and prurient interest that this field quickly attracted.[2]

But endocrinology achieved some medical respectability and scientific acclaim by about 1901, when scientists J. J. Abel and Jokichi Takamine at Johns Hopkins University isolated epinephrine, the hormone of the adrenal gland responsible for raising blood pressure. The Parke-Davis drug firm marketed it successfully as Adrenalin (especially valuable when injected locally for reducing surgical bleeding). In 1917, E. C. Kendall at the Mayo Clinic isolated from the thyroid gland a substance he called thyroxine, a major hormone involved in regulating metabolism. By the time the First World War ended, biochemists and endocrinologists worldwide were feverishly working to purify and understand the natural hormones produced by the testes and ovaries, the pancreas, the pituitary gland, and essentially all the other glands thought to modulate physiological functions. Endocrinologists took decades to work out all the details, but researchers already understood that these substances acted as powerful chemical signals throughout the body. The triumphant isolation of insulin by Frederick Banting and Charles Best at the University of Toronto and its subsequent marketing in the early 1920s by the Lilly firm saved the lives of millions of diabetics and brought enormous luster to the hormone field.[3]

Doctors' embrace of glandular understandings of disease opened a new market for hormonal treatments. Following the lead of Parke-Davis and Lilly, numerous pharmaceutical manufacturers began sponsoring hormone research in hopes of obtaining exclusive rights to a marketable preparation based on a leading endocrinologist's work. By the late 1920s, drug companies' enthusiasm for hormone research had created a "gold rush" in endocrinology.[4]

As endocrinology's status rose in the 1920s, it claimed obesity as its intellectual and commercial terrain. Several now-rare frank disorders of the thyroid and pituitary glands were particularly important in establishing this connection. In the early twentieth century, many children still suffered what was then called cretinism, a syndrome of retarded mental development and growth that had in the late nineteenth century been linked to insufficient iodine in the diet. One symptom of cretinism is the presence of goiter (a swollen thyroid gland in the neck), which led to the discovery that iodine is normally concentrated in the thyroid and that the gland secretes an iodine-containing hormone. Myxedema, a general term meaning thyroid insufficiency, was also more common at that time in adults than at present. Its many symptoms, along with goiter, include low heart rate, low blood pressure, depressed metabolic rate, feelings of lethargy and depression, and weight gain. Somewhat similarly, the very rare condition (then and now) called Froelich syndrome involves retarded sexual and mental development, low blood pressure, obesity, and sometimes also abnormal fat distribution, but not typically thyroid enlargement. Discovered in association with brain tumors, Froelich syndrome helped lead to the understanding that the pituitary gland produces a hormone that regulates the thyroid gland's own hormone production along with hormones affecting growth and gonads. Since these serious diseases involve hormones and affect weight, many endocrinologists believed that common fatness was also due to glandular disturbances affecting the thyroid, albeit more subtly. In 1924, San Francisco endocrinologist Hans Lisser confidently asserted to a friendly audience that not even "50 percent of obesity is entirely exogenous" (caused by overeating alone). Instead, he explained, most cases involve another "factor," that is, "an abnormal faulty metabolism the control of which is to a large extent dominated by the glands of internal secretion."[5]

A tongue-in-cheek 1927 commentary by one physician about another shows the extent to which hormones had saturated the medical imagination, at least concerning body type:

> The physician who knows something about the ductless glands and what they do
> in the way of fashioning the human body needs no one to talk to him as he walks

down the street. There is no better sport for such a man than picking out the ductless gland types as he walks along. . . .

First there was a father 6 feet tall, weighing 145 pounds. His hands were long, slender, and artistic. His feet were long and slender. His build was supposed to indicate a moderately active anterior lobe of his pituitary.

His wife was 4 feet 11 inches tall. She had hands typical of anterior lobe insufficiency. They had short, broad palms and short, tapering fingers. Her body showed girdle obesity. These characteristics indicated deficiency of the posterior lobe of the pituitary. Her skin was cold and alabaster white with a flushing of her cheeks. She had padding of the backs of her hands and feet and of her neck just above the collar bone. Her hair was scanty. Her metabolic rate was low. These qualities showed she had a thyroid deficiency in addition to her other [pituitary] deficiency.

The oldest daughter is 5 feet 2 inches and heavy. Her obesity is of the girdle type. Her short stature, delicate frame, and small hands and feet indicate preadolescent deficiency of the anterior pituitary.[6]

This style of impressionistic diagnosis was especially popular among doctors treating childhood obesity, writes historian Laura Dawes. Pediatricians employed diagnostic rules of thumb like "[fatty] hips-means-gonads / shoulders-means-thyroid." While today the practice seems as archaic as phrenology, these doctors could point to expert opinions in support of their extrapolations about hormones and body fat.[7]

While the latest lab research concerning the glands doubtless helped to make such thinking plausible for doctors and patients, the linkage between the thyroid gland and obesity was forged more by practical opportunity than scientific theory. Dessicated beef or pork thyroids, available as medicines since the early 1900s, raise the heart rate and metabolic rate when consumed, and purer preparations that could be injected were available in the 1920s. Whether or not an overweight patient's metabolism was actually slow or her thyroid hormone levels actually deficient—niceties very seldom tested by physicians—thyroid drugs resulted in weight loss.

Thyroid-powered weight loss gained popularity quickly. Endocrinology's contribution to diabetes care notwithstanding, by the 1930s the field had become known jokingly among physicians as the specialty "primarily concerned with making fat ladies thin."[8] The comfortable incomes of endocrine specialists drew on the cultural currency of the glands, the commercial availability of hormone drugs (especially powdered thyroid preparations), and, of course, the steady supply of patients wishing to be thinner. Indeed, thanks to fashion and beauty trends favoring slimness,

1929 Belles Are Not Fat

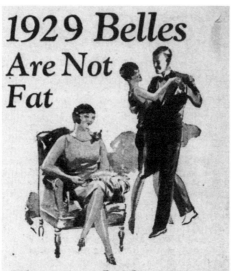

They end the excess in this easy way

Twenty years ago excess fat was common. Few people of 40 escaped it. Not so today. Slender figures are the rule. All ideas of style and beauty are opposed to fat.

This great change started when science discovered the chief cause of obesity. It lies in an under-active gland. A way was found to correct this deficiency, and multitudes employed it.

This factor was embodied in Marmola prescription tablets. People have used them for over 20 years—millions of boxes of them. That is one great reason for the slender figures you see everywhere today.

Marmola is not secret. Each box contains the formula and the reasons for results. No abnormal exercise or diet is required. Simply take four tablets daily until weight comes down to normal.

Try this method if you over-weigh. Watch the new health and vigor which come when the excess fat departs. Then you will know why so many people, for many years, have urged friends to use Marmola. Go start at once.

Marmola prescription tablets are sold by all druggists at $1 per box. If your druggist is out, he will get them at once from his jobber.

MARMOLA
Prescription Tablets
The Pleasant Way to Reduce

Advertisement for Marmola thyroid-and-laxative weight-loss pills, sold by prescription and directly to consumers, emphasized thyroid gland deficiency as the cause of obesity. Source: *Baltimore Sun*, January 27, 1929, 61.

insurance firms found that female policyholders—that is, mainly women of the middle and upper classes—lost on average three to five pounds for their heights during the 1920s.[9] Physicians like Lisser prescribed a treatment regimen that might last anywhere between four months and several years, which mostly consisted of taking thyroid pills to maintain a constantly elevated metabolic rate. Some specialists prescribed sex hormones or pituitary hormones; some required their patients to see them weekly.[10]

Like all gold rushes, the glandular gold rush ended quickly. By the late 1930s physicians had both scientific and clinical reasons for retreating from endocrinological explanations of obesity. First, medical authorities began to see thyroid gland powders and extracts as dangerous quackery. Thyroid hormones' powerful effects on the heart can cause toxicity and death. These reactions were in fact commonly seen among people who took the drug just to lose weight, since they generally had no other symptoms (other than fatness) of actual thyroid hormone deficiency or metabolic deficiency. In the 1920s, endocrinologists shrugged off these potential side effects; Lisser assured his physician listeners that "many obese patients have a normal metabolic rate, and despite this fact can sometimes tolerate large doses of thyroid extract without toxic symptoms and without raising it above normal."[11] But with use of the drug becoming more widespread in the 1930s, often by individuals trying to lose weight without a doctor's help, more and more people were being poisoned.

Finally in 1937, after a decade-long campaign, federal authorities moved to shut down the leading nonprescription vendor, the Raladam firm of Detroit. Raladam heavily advertised its Marmola product in newspapers and ladies magazines with extravagant claims, for example that excess fat "simply slips away" without strict dieting or backbreaking exercise. Typically mentioning "glands" but not thyroid hormones explicitly, the ads correctly claimed that Marmola "contains the same element prescribed by most doctors in treating their fat patients."[12] The rationale given by the Federal Trade Commission in 1937 was that "based on distinguished medical and scientific opinion . . . only a small proportion of cases of over-weight result from thyroid deficiency; that in many cases the respondent company's product cannot be safely used, and in any case should be taken only on the advice of a physician." (That Marmola contained more laxative than thyroid hormone seems to have been a less powerful argument.) In 1938 the Food and Drug Administration (FDA) helped suppress Marmola and imitator products by declaring thyroid hormones to be available only by prescription, one of the first actions the agency took after gaining new powers to govern drug safety.[13]

The government's explanation of its decision to prohibit nonprescription sales of thyroid hormones points to the second reason that endocrinology fell out of favor as a rationale for fatness: an emerging scientific consensus that overweight and obesity, except in extremely rare cases, had nothing to do with metabolic rates or with hormones that regulate metabolism. One of the key researchers in this area was L. H. Newburgh, an influential physiologist at the University of Michigan. In the 1930s Newburgh conducted a series of experiments with volunteers, human guinea pigs who were subjected to the discomfort of long days on a respirometer or were shut inside the cabinets used to measure metabolism precisely at the time. His studies showed that when all the material consumed and excreted by people is carefully accounted for, fat people and thin people have about the same basal or resting metabolic rates (proportional to body surface area). Certainly, there are deviations from the average, but some thin people have below-average metabolic rates, and some fat people have above-average rates. Newburgh additionally showed that certain prior findings taken as evidence that obesity arises from metabolic derangement, such as weight gain among overweight people on a reducing diet, were due to water uptake or measurement error.[14]

Newburgh's findings can be summarized concisely: fatter people get that way simply because they eat more. As he put the emerging mainstream view in one prominent 1930 research report, in the majority of obese people, "the laying on of fat is the outcome of a perverted habit." These people either "require stimuli of greater intensity before they feel satisfied; or else they deliberately disregard the warning in order to continue a little longer the pleasures that come with eating." In some cases, this is a learned behavior, adopted at the behest of overeager parents and open to correction. But others, he warned, cannot help themselves. In these people, "the combination of weak will and a pleasure-seeking outlook upon life, lays the background for the condition." These are the addicts, whose condition "resembles that of the chronic alcoholics."[15]

Newburgh acknowledged that there are those who become overweight because they genuinely suffer from one of the rare endocrine disorders that reduces the basal metabolic rate, but they are the rare exception. Newburgh's intuition that obesity is mainly caused by a psychiatric perversion akin to alcoholism or due to poor parenting (or both) would soon be embraced by the fields of psychiatry and medicine. The newspapers, meanwhile, immediately grasped the implications of his metabolic work for the moral status of fat people: "Just Gluttony Makes Obesity— Michigan Professor Strips Defense of Portly."[16]

An Emerging Stigma

Well before the FDA banned their sale, over-the-counter thyroid pills developed a reputation for dangerous and unpleasant side effects. They produced a racing heart, palpitations, sweating, and diarrhea, and, used improperly, they could cause a heart attack. That many patients tolerated, and even sought, such treatment reflects the harsh penalties of being fat. This had not always been the case. According to social historians, fatness in the West had traditionally been a fairly uncommon condition found mainly among the wealthy, and it was positively regarded as a sign of robust health and good humor. Nineteenth-century medical textbooks urged doctors to counsel dietary restraint in cases of gross obesity but otherwise suggested no forceful intervention.[17]

Societal attitudes about fatness in the United States began to shift dramatically around the turn of the twentieth century. With industrialization and urbanization, fatness emerged in the popular imagination as an unseemly marker of laziness and intemperate appetite. Beginning around 1890, new, morally loaded descriptors for fatness appeared in general use, such as the phrase "fat slob." Advertisements for slimming foods, underclothes, and gadgets became common in newspaper advertising. At the same time, medical professionals came to regard obesity as a serious danger to health. And life insurance companies began penalizing overweight customers for their elevated risk of premature mortality.[18]

This new stigma fell particularly hard on women. Women's fashions in the 1920s began to glamorize an especially slim figure, and home weighing scales became more common. The health and beauty columns of major newspapers during this time were replete with dieting advice, and there were frequent references to the fashion of "exaggerated slimness" (conjured partly with long, snug skirts or trousers and high heels). Weight-loss products capitalized on the trend: as one Marmola ad put it, "1929 Belles Are Not Fat"—and thanks to science's discovery that "the chief cause of obesity . . . lies in an under-active gland," nobody needed to be.[19] The new fashions were themselves a reaction to the new moral significance of fatness as a mark of culpable failure in self-control. As sociologist Amy Erdman Farrell has argued, suffragettes strove to maintain slim figures so as to demonstrate their self-control, maturity, and responsibility—in short, their fitness for political rights. Women responded to this pressure by seeking medical treatment. Of the thirty obesity patients Lisser described as representative of his practice in the mid-1920s, twenty-six were women. The "fat lady" jibe about endocrinologists was not far off target.[20]

Thus, on top of their struggle to meet beauty standards, people perceived as fat faced outright repugnance. An exchange between syndicated advice and beauty columnist Antoinette Donnelly and a reader was unusual only for its bluntness. When the reader asked why women should lose weight despite frequent warnings to avoid dietary and medical fads, Donnelly responded that "fat is ugly," "unhealthy," and "not entitled to the easy tolerance it is often met with" because it is mainly caused by "inactivity," "overeating," and "wrong eating"—that is, indolence, self-indulgence, and perverse appetites. "Why Be a Stodgy Fat Vegetable When You Can Be a Flower?," she asked her readers.[21] Many similar expressions of disdain can be found in the media of the 1920s and 1930s.

Donnelly did make an exception for those whose fatness could be explained by a genuine glandular disorder. In this context, the appeal of such a glandular diagnosis is clear. But when scientists began to question the link between hormones and obesity, the mainstream media turned on those who had sought shelter in thyroid treatments.[22] By the second half of the 1930s, newspapers expressed increased skepticism about hormonal explanations of obesity. Articles began to suggest that glands were merely an "excuse" with which the fat disguised their "gluttony." By 1940, even medical proponents of the hormonal "alibi" agreed with critics that more than 98 percent of adult "fatties" were overweight strictly because of overeating and inactivity (though some held out for a higher percentage of glandular disorders among overweight children).[23]

That obesity is caused by overeating was an issue on which medical experts and beauty columnists could for once agree. This consensus, however, led to a more contentious question: Why do fat people overeat?

The Overprotected Child

The thinker most responsible for replacing the endocrinological paradigm for obesity with a psychological one studied children, not adults: the young German-trained pediatrician Hilde Bruch of Babies Hospital, an institution affiliated with Columbia University. In 1935 Bruch was put in charge of the new outpatient Vanderbilt Clinic for endocrine disorders, which mainly handled children referred by school nurses and others for suspected "glandular problems." Given that she had no training in psychiatry, she might have been expected to simply continue the line of treatment being proposed at the clinic. After a suicide attempt later in 1935, however, Bruch began psychotherapy with Gotthard Booth, a psychiatrist who, like her, had recently arrived from Germany in the wake of the Nazi takeover. She would

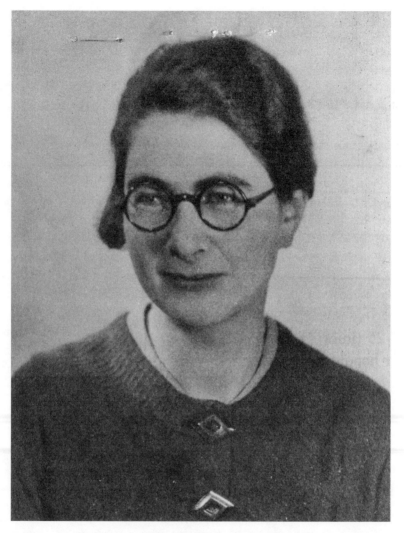

Pediatrician and psychiatrist Hilde Bruch, 1941. Courtesy of Rockefeller Archive Center.

continue in therapy for many years, and this personal contact with psychiatry evidently stimulated her professional interest in the field where she would make her greatest mark—ultimately undermining the rationale for the clinic where she worked.[24]

Bruch recalled that the fat children she saw in the endocrine clinic often behaved differently from the children in the rest of her clinical experience. As she described in an account written several years later, these children often took the only chair in the examining room (other than the doctor's) "while the mother stood." They would remain seated, "with the mother's approval," even when Bruch suggested that the child let the mother sit. In general, these overweight children seemed accustomed to being "waited on" by the parent. Thus Bruch began to feel "there was something very wrong with the way the mothers treated these children." She began to suspect that the family, rather than the glands, lay behind the obese child's problems.[25]

Bruch began to document this mother-blaming hunch. She carefully measured the fat children's various body parts, took X-rays to assess their level of skeletal maturation, and, when possible, obtained birth and other medical records. Of more than a hundred prepubescent children she examined over a period of two and a half years at the Vanderbilt Clinic, nearly all—excluding those with mental deficiency, which can be a sign of a marked thyroid deficiency (cretinism)—were above average in height for their age, and most were also more advanced in skeletal maturity. They were not abnormally large at birth, however. These findings challenged the common view that fatness resulted from pituitary or thyroid hormone deficiencies, since either of these conditions slows physical development in children. Also, those children who had been receiving endocrinological treatment seemed unresponsive to it. One six-year-old boy, for example, had already received more than a hundred injections of pituitary hormone but remained 50 percent overweight (at eighty pounds). Bruch concluded that the fatness of these children was best explained by supposing that they simply ate more than their thinner peers.[26]

A paper that Bruch published in 1939 based on such evidence was just one among an impressive sheaf of reports she published during a two-year interval, which (together with Newburgh's) collectively dealt a deadly blow to the glandular perspective.[27] Having put a final nail in the coffin of the theory that obesity is mainly a metabolic problem, Bruch recommended that researchers turn their attention to family structure and socialization. In another paper, for instance, she surveyed the parents of the fat children she saw, asking whether they had friends to play with regularly and about their level of physical activity. Although the study lacked a control group of non-obese children from the same population, she found that the fat children who had friends were much more likely to be physically active than those without. She interpreted these data as evidence that social maladjustment played a role in the physical inactivity of fat children, which supported her overall view that children (and adults) become fat simply because they eat more food than they use

up through basal metabolism and exercise. Thus, she supposed, fat children without friends would be less likely to escape adult obesity than those with friends who
engaged them in active play. This same study reported that 70 percent of the fat
children were the youngest sibling or the only child and were treated overprotec-
tively as the "baby" of the family. Many of these children seemed to lack basic skills:
even ten-year-olds relied on their parents to get dressed and undressed.[28]

A third paper described Bruch's efforts to learn how much food the obese children were eating. Bruch acknowledged that surveying and interviewing overweight
children (or their parents) about what they ate each day was unlikely to yield accurate reports of her patients' diets. Nevertheless, she made an interesting discovery
about parental attitudes during the process. More than two-thirds of the parents
reported that their children had unusually strong ("good," "tremendous," "vora-
cious") appetites. The parents were proud of how much their fat children ate.[29] Here
and elsewhere, Bruch explored the insight that it was psychology, not physiology,
that made these children fat.

Bruch's efforts to understand her patients' family situations took her to their
homes; this work in some ways paralleled community health surveys, albeit on a
smaller scale. In a collaboration with social worker Grace Touraine, Bruch visited
the homes of forty representative children from her clinic. Each researcher separately interviewed the mother and, when possible, the father. Many of the obese
children's families were quite poor, but their homes were unusually well kept—
even immaculate. Frequently, Bruch and Touraine found that the children had been
allotted only a small space, if any at all, for active or creative play out of fear that
their actions might disorganize or harm the furnishings. Many families had grand-
parents or other relatives living with them in the small apartments, further con-
straining the children and exposing them to mixed signals. "On the one hand," the
authors wrote, "the children were deprived of needed space, and nagged and hushed
constantly. On the other hand central guidance was lacking, and the children were
exposed to 'spoiling' and to controversies and discussions over their rearing." Despite the marginal economic status of these families, they complained about the
cost of everything except food. Their budgets prioritized ample home-cooked meals
"disproportionately . . . as compared to money available for other needs of the child,
such as clothing or tools and equipment for play and athletics."[30]

Bruch and Touraine put the blame for this situation squarely on the mothers.
Their complaints against these women ranged from charges of self-pity to rejecting
their children. The mothers' typical main failing was an inconsistency: their "overt

display of protectiveness[,] . . . devotion and affection . . . barely covered the underlying insecurity in relation to the child," which was often laced with guilt from not wanting the child. Overcontrolling and overprotective, the mothers would not let their children play outside or do anything potentially risky. Rather, they squashed their children's initiative by continuing to do everything for them as they had since the child's earliest years. Instead of offering reliable emotional support—they often addressed their children with irritation and treated them harshly—they expressed love by feeding and performing services for the children.[31]

Somewhat paradoxically, given how these mothers discouraged their children from taking initiative, the parents had high ambitions for their kids. But with so few avenues for self-expression available, these unfortunate children ate as a form of performance that brought reliable rewards. Having now embraced the lexicon of midcentury psychology, Bruch wrote, "The obese child, impeded in the dynamic expression of his self, manifests his creative strivings in the static form of bodily largeness. The inordinate expansion reveals the inmost desire of the child to be big and powerful."[32] Lacking the opportunity to play with other children their age, such fat children fell further and further behind in motor and social skills. Then, the swelling bulk of the child would solidify his or her status as a social outcast. A self-reinforcing pattern of pursuing satisfaction through eating instead of through outward, active challenges would be established well before puberty. The fat child, Bruch suggested, clings to a baby's pattern of satisfaction and sets himself on the path to becoming a lonely, underachieving obese adult.[33]

Bruch had no formal training in psychiatry when she wrote these seminal papers. In 1941, she moved to Baltimore to study psychiatry at Johns Hopkins University with funding from the Rockefeller Foundation. She initially worked with the famed discoverer of autism, Leo Kanner (no orthodox Freudian), and she also began seeing the noted psychoanalyst Frieda Fromm-Reichmann for therapy. Perhaps Bruch's unconventional, indirect introduction to psychoanalytic thinking through her own therapy and her friendships with eclectic and iconoclast psychoanalysts at Columbia, including Helen Flanders Dunbar, explains Bruch's enduring, unusually broad interest in family dynamics. For Bruch, the interesting question was the relationship between food, family conflict, and assertive action in the face of repressed self-expression. Because of its complex origins, obesity could almost be regarded as a cultural disease. But despite Bruch's nuanced thought, for much of American medicine any psychological explanation of overeating began and ended with the Freudian concept of oral fixation.[34]

Food, the Essential Addiction

When other psychiatrists learned of Bruch's work, they immediately saw the potential of applying orthodox Freudian notions of sexual development to the phenomenon of obesity. By the 1940s Freudian psychoanalysis had gained dominance in American psychiatry and was well positioned to benefit from psychiatric medicine's new postwar importance. According to Freud, infants developed according to a fixed series of stages, minor variations in which explained their adult character. Initially the infant's experience is dominated by uncomfortable hunger and its pleasurable satisfaction at the breast—the oral stage. As the child develops physical awareness, it enters the anal stage where pain and pleasure revolve around defecation and its control. Then, as it becomes more sexually aware, it desires the parent of the opposite sex but is frustrated, entering the Oedipal crisis, which when resolved eventually leads to the final, genital stage—a healthy interest in heterosexual intercourse outside the family. While the American psychoanalytic church included its share of dissidents and heretics, some deviating in their interpretation of the canonical stages, these ideas had broad currency in psychiatry and beyond.[35] Certainly, most American doctors were acquainted with the general developmental scheme, including the concept of oral fixation. This is a disorder or defect in an adult reflecting (partial) developmental arrest at the oral stage, in which abnormally great energy goes to pursuing satisfaction by oral consumption. Once pointed out, the connection between overeating and orality seemed obvious, and over the next decade orality became the general explanation for other perversions of consumption, including alcoholism and smoking.[36]

A paper delivered by Cleveland psychiatrist George Reeve at a 1942 psychiatric meeting is a typical early example of this thinking. Citing Bruch and psychoanalyst Franz Alexander as authorities, Reeve considered it established that obesity "is related to gaining oral satisfaction."[37] The patient group he described consisted of women who had become obese in young adulthood. One woman showed "marked psychoneurotic manifestations relating to competition with her sister for attention of their father," for whom "eating [became] a compensation for frustrated libido, and also a 'reason' for not leaving home." Another used eating as a "direct defense mechanism" in that she ate "huge quantities of food and candy" whenever "a suitor became very interested and attentive," only to quickly lose weight again when the "suitor became disgusted and left." A third, married, whose "husband's ideal woman is slender," was "frigid" and ate aggressively in "defiance of the husband's wishes." Another married woman ate uncontrollably, despite the fact that this filled her with self-loathing; she saw excess "eating as 'immoral' and . . . a substitution for sex relations," and she perceived "a connection between her desire for meat, her interest in sausage and 'her masculine wishes.'" According to Reeve, all these fat women "gained emotional satisfactions from their eating" instead of from mature genital fulfillment, some using it aggressively or sadistically, some defensively, some perhaps masochistically.[38]

Another early adopter was Henry Richardson, a New York physician and psychotherapist who hoped to fully integrate "psychiatric knowledge of oral drives and passive receptive trends" into the interpretation of obesity. In describing the case of one overweight, successful school principal, who underwent therapy for depression with him during the early 1940s, he reported that the middle-aged woman had a childhood characterized by an unloving and domineering mother and a warmer but distant father. Much like Bruch's typical obese child, Richardson's patient learned to substitute food for the parental love that she lacked. Diverging somewhat from Bruch, Richardson went on to interpret the development of his patient's neurosis into adulthood, showing how her parents suppressed her knowledge of sex throughout adolescence, how the resolution of her "Oedipal situation" was frustrated by her father's early death, and ultimately how her fatness had become both a defense against and a substitute for sexuality. By gaining bulk, this patient was expressing her urge to become pregnant strictly "by way of the gastrointestinal tract."[39] But other than a more explicit interpretation of orality in the light of mature psychosexual development, there is little in Richardson's account that differs from Bruch's concept of obesity, which he credited as "foundational."

Oral fixation took on a similar but deeper significance as the key to understanding all kinds of addiction—including obesity—in the work of psychiatrist Otto Fenichel. In his 1945 *Psychoanalytic Theory of Neurosis*, which became the standard American medical textbook on neuroses during the early postwar era, Fenichel classified many "impulse neuroses and perversions" as addictive disorders caused by oral fixation. According to Fenichel, all addicts are people who never stably matured to the genital stage. Predisposed through an "archaic oral longing," the irresistible consumption of a substance experienced "as food and warmth" causes addicts to degenerate toward the primitive "oral orientation of the infant." Fenichel's explicit comparison of the obese to narcotic addicts—"junkies" in the parlance of the time—was a damning diagnosis. Nothing could be more unflattering in the mid-twentieth-century United States, where addiction represented such dangerous deviance that drug users were routinely locked away for years in federal prisons merely for drug possession.[40]

Fenichel acknowledged that not all fat people fit this oral fixation model perfectly. For the less degenerate obese neurotics, eating might be a perverse form of excess activity used to master periodic guilt, anxiety, or depression. In the same way that other neurotics used excess exercise or work to combat stress, these over-eaters used food as a coping mechanism. Fenichel made another exception for the depressive or bipolar individual (always female) for whom eating represents a hostile, "oral-sadistic" struggle with or attack on the mother. In language similar to that used by Reeve and Richardson, Fenichel described this sadistic, unresolved-Oedipal type of overeater as someone who substituted a defiant eating binge for sex—an attractive but frightening "dirty meal." Sausages exemplified the food of choice for this class of binging woman.[41]

A number of other psychiatric thinkers explored variations on these themes. In 1950, for instance, Gustav Bychowski offered a supposedly original psychoanalytic theory of obesity that combined the oral fixation concept with the ego defense concept. In Bychowski's theory, fatness constitutes a regressed or primitive somatic or "autoplastic" reaction to Oedipal conflicts, whereas a mature "alloplastic reaction" would confront, challenge, and remake the external situation instead of the body. For the fat women he psychoanalyzed, food was not just a vehicle for oral gratification, but also an attempt to incorporate and "impersonate both the breast and the phallus." Surprisingly, Bychowski here neglected to discuss sausages.[42]

All of this suggests how quickly the idea of obesity as a form of oral fixation—often attributed to Bruch despite her avoidance of the term—permeated American psychiatric thinking about mental health. Although it did spare the patient from hormone injections, the new medical understanding was far less forgiving to fat people. By the 1940s, even some endocrinologically inclined doctors were incorporating psychiatric theories into their practice. During that decade, for example, Philadelphia thyroid specialist and family practitioner Israel Bram, in tune with current views that obesity rarely reflected thyroid deficiency, subjected more than 1,000 of his overweight patients to a tough-talking program of "simple psychotherapy and dietetic discipline." Bram understood their fatness as a psychosomatic expression of escapist oral compensation for failure to master the "worries and tensions of existence."[43]

One astonishing sign of the reach of psychodynamic theories about obesity during this time is an observation by the sociologist David Riesman in his 1950 classic, *The Lonely Crowd*. Based on his extensive interviews with American children and adults across the social spectrum during the 1940s, Riesman reported that "upper middle-class parents are becoming hesitant to tell children to eat something because it is good for them—lest they create oral complexes."[44]

A Cold War Character Flaw

Bruch chose the right time for her advocacy of mental explanations of obesity. One factor contributing to psychiatry's greatly elevated status and influence was the unprecedented role of psychiatrists in the Second World War. Leading psychiatrists advised military planners at an early stage on how to reduce manpower losses due to so-called shell shock, a massive problem of the First World War. Psychiatrists also screened recruits, designed training materials for inducted soldiers, and once the fighting began established effective methods for treating what came to be called "combat fatigue" on the front lines (but was termed "war neurosis" and "psychoneurotic breakdown" when the psychiatrists spoke to each other).[45]

Psychiatrists eagerly applied the lessons they had learned with the military to the rest of the American population. Based on the percentage of draftees rejected on psychiatric grounds, it became a recognized "fact" in postwar medical discourse that 10 percent of Americans suffered from some form of mental illness. The widely publicized crisis of the asylums, according to which "every other bed" in the nation's hospital system was occupied by a psychiatric patient, stressed the urgent need to do more about the nation's mental health. In 1946, Congress passed the National Mental Health Act, establishing the National Institute of Mental Health (NIMH) under the NIH's growing umbrella of medical research institutes. Although it would take Congress two more years to fund the NIMH, the fact that the institute was established at all, officially ahead of the Heart Institute that would address the top national cause of death, speaks to the cultural and political importance of psychiatry in postwar American thinking about health.[46]

Once the Cold War began at the end of the 1940s, psychiatry took on even greater importance as an instrument to reinforce the nuclear family—the country's primary fortification against communism. As mental health advocate Charles Schlaifer argued before Congress in a successful 1953 appeal to boost the NIMH's funding, "It is no accident that in the dictatorship countries, in Hitler's Germany and in Stalin's Russia, psychiatry as we practice it in America has been rejected." "We know," Schlaifer continued, "that the vigor and mental health of the American family is the greatest bulwark against turning to subversive activity and juvenile delinquency and drug addiction . . . and all the other problems that walk arm in arm with mental illness in its various forms."[47] This kind of thinking had a plausibility in the early postwar era that is hard today to conceive.

With mental health looming large in concerns about social stability and national security, psychiatric explanations of misbehavior, unhappiness, and even simple nonconformity became cultural commonplaces from advice columns to Broadway shows (such as the 1957 hit *West Side Story*, in which a delinquent blames "society" for his crimes). Psychiatrists and popular commentators alike expressed particular concern about correcting the neuroses of women because, according to psychoanalytic theory, inappropriate mothering was causing mental disorders in the next generation of Americans. This logic helps to explain the massive midcentury drugging of middle-class women with tranquilizers and antidepressant stimulants at the hands of their doctors.[48] Even psychologists who rejected Freudian strictures gained popularity in the Cold War context. As Americans looked homeward to domestic life for security and satisfaction in a threatening atomic world, they embraced emotional fulfillment as their highest goal.[49] Bruch's account of obesity as the result of an unhappy childhood and poor mothering meshed perfectly with the tone of the times.

This psychiatry-happy cultural context helps explain why the popular press welcomed the news that overweight people were driven to overeat by "subconscious" "emotions" and abnormal "mental cravings." Women's magazines and advice columnists found the psychological theory of fatness based on sexual development to be irresistible. One columnist counseled that the best cure is to "recognize your insecurity" and "seek the basic cause" to lessen your "emotional dependence on food" and identify "what can be changed by your own efforts." In short, fat women should "learn to act like grownups." Another advice column in 1947, referencing Richardson's work on obesity in women, was headlined "If You're Too Plump, Girls, Stop Being Afraid of Men."[50] The new medical understanding of obesity, rooted in psychoanalysis, also fit well with the established popular stigma that fatness was a moral failing and a character flaw. That stigma now merged, through oral fixation theory, with that surrounding other kinds of addiction as a craven retreat from life's adult challenges. But the stain of obesity was more gendered than the other moral failings, and authorities particularly excoriated fat women as threats to heterosexuality, motherhood, and ultimately the nation's sanity and fighting strength.

Yet psychiatry had not quite finished finding the character flaws associated with fatness. In the later 1940s and into the 1950s, the view emerged that not only had fat people suffered especially unhappy childhoods and in general showed pronounced "emotional tension" or neurosis, but they were often victims of deeper emotional illness who were attempting to manage their condition through eating.[51] One advocate of this point of view was a psychiatrist based in Rochester, New York, with the memorable name of W. W. Hamburger. While Hamburger acknowledged that some obese people ate in an escapist, addiction-like retreat from challenges or in a perversion of sexual impulses, he found that others exhibited a much less direct relation between their problem and its expression than "orality" would imply. These patients turned to overeating to manage a serious underlying depression (or, less often, hysteria), drawing on the positive emotional associations people develop with food through childhood as a survival strategy. Many children, for example, are offered ice cream as a reward for good behavior; as adults, Hamburger's patients turned to ice cream for the feelings of approval and self-esteem it conjured as an alternative to abject despair. For fat patients in this category, Hamburger argued, it was more important to understand and treat the depression than to make them stop overeating, since removing food would effectively kick away their crutches and worsen their mental state.[52] Similarly, the influential Philadelphia psychiatrist Albert Stunkard found that many obese people reacted passively to negative or depressing events, decreasing their calorie-consuming physical activity in situations where healthy people reacted by increasing activity. From this more behavioral perspective, Stunkard described a situation in which setbacks in life produced both depression and obesity.[53]

All of these stigmatizing themes—obesity as a deviance from heterosexual maturity, as a failure of adult willpower akin to alcoholism and narcotic addiction, and as a sign of a serious depressive disorder marked by passivity and withdrawal, along with the special concern with mothers' mental health as a keystone of democracy in the Cold War—had merged in the medical imagination by the early 1950s. The pharmaceutical industry recognized this, and it was reflected in advertising campaigns for prescription diet pills. Indeed, the drug firms' use of these themes in marketing their products to physicians must have cemented this view of obesity among medical professionals. Doctors' interactions with their patients then reinforced the message that the general population was seeing in the popular press, including advice columns.

The Diet Pill Bonanza

When thyroid hormone lost its legitimacy as a weight-loss treatment in the late 1930s, doctors needed a new tool. They soon found it in amphetamine and closely related drugs. Amphetamine had not originally been marketed as a weight-loss medication. The original amphetamine was invented in the late 1920s as a decongestant that might improve on the performance of adrenaline and the successful plant-derived compound ephedrine, to which it was similar chemically. Marketed from the mid-1930s by the Smith, Kline and French (SKF) drug firm under the brand name Benzedrine, amphetamine achieved some commercial success as a decongestant, especially in inhaler form. But it soon achieved greater success and acclaim in pill form as the first "antidepressant."

By the late 1930s physicians had a high regard for Benzedrine, which they enthusiastically began to prescribe as a psychiatric drug. Many of them saw it as almost a magic bullet—the first pill that allowed them specifically to "affect, even create, mood" and thereby open "inexhaustible" "possibilities . . . in the therapeutic care of neuropsychiatric disorders."[54] With the postwar rise of psychiatry both as a medical specialty and as a broader concern for American society, psychiatric prescriptions for Benzedrine skyrocketed, as did prescriptions for its new sister product from SKF, Dexedrine (boasting a lower side-effect profile). Unsurprisingly, SKF encouraged this trend through heavy advertising to family doctors as well as psychiatrists, urging them to recognize and treat previously overlooked neuroses with amphetamine. Close on SKF's heels, competing firms like Lilly and Abbott marketed copycat pills for the same uses but based on methamphetamine, which is pharmacologically almost indistinguishable from amphetamine but was unprotected by patents (because its adrenaline-like effects had been discovered and described decades before by Japanese scientists).[55]

In Benzedrine's first decade on the market, SKF did not promote it as a diet drug. During the war, however, the company learned that large quantities of diet pills containing amphetamine, sometimes mixed with thyroid hormones, were being manufactured by small fly-by-night firms. The companies sold the drugs at a fraction of Benzedrine's price to questionable diet doctors, who dispensed them directly to their patients at great profit. The weight-loss specialists understood that combining the hormonal effects of the thyroid extract with the mood-lifting effects of amphetamine helped their patients lose weight and feel happier. Furthermore, amphetamine seemed to suppress appetite quite apart from its mood effects, as SKF had been aware from the drug's earliest clinical trials.[56] But SKF had seen more promise in its patented new product as a psychiatric medicine.

In the mid-twentieth century, drug companies did not need government permission to market a product to doctors as useful for some particular medical condition. But if they wished to advertise in the major medical journals, the most influential vehicle for reaching prescribing doctors, they needed to convince the American Medical Association's Council on Pharmacy and Chemistry (from 1957, it was called the Council on Drugs) that their advertising claims were well supported by evidence. A company would commission studies of a drug's safety and efficacy from reputable scientists and clinicians and submit the results for the council's review. If this elite panel of pharmacologists and other experts accepted the results, the AMA would issue a seal of approval that allowed manufacturers to advertise the drug for particular uses in the journals (almost all of which cooperated). The fly-by-night amphetamine makers did not have this approval and marketed directly to diet doctors and pharmacists. SKF had quietly initiated controlled studies on amphetamine as a weight-loss drug during the war, but the company held back on applying for council permission to advertise it as such, fearing that AMA approval would only benefit their shady competitors. In 1947, however, after federal courts confirmed SKF's patent on Benzedrine, the company swung into action. To avoid expensive infringement litigation, the small competitors switched their formulas to methamphetamine, while SKF moved into the diet pill business with its respected Benzedrine brand, applying for and receiving approval to advertise it for weight loss later that year.[57]

Thus, amphetamine, already a highly acclaimed psychiatric drug, started being heavily marketed to doctors as a diet pill just when the psychiatric account of obesity was achieving dominance in medical and popular understanding. Even so, the first wave of SKF advertising for Benzedrine (and Dexedrine) as a weight-loss treatment omitted reference to psychiatric themes. The initial medical journal advertisements took a conservative line, simply stressing that experts now condemned the use of thyroid hormones for weight loss but endorsed amphetamine as safe and effective. One full-page advertisement that ran in the *Journal of the American Medical Association* and other general medicine journals in 1948 and 1949, for example, is entitled "For Medically Sound Reduction of Overweight." The main copy draws a contrast between "Benzedrine Sulfate—rational and accepted" and "Thyroid—irrational, potentially dangerous and widely condemned." Smaller text explains that SKF's amphetamine product "safely depresses the overweight patient's appetite" and thus reduces her weight without affecting basal metabolic rate, heart rate, or blood pressure. Thyroid, on the other hand, adversely affects all of these and is strongly condemned by "most authorities," "except in those rare instances when an accompanying hypothyroidism has been definitely demonstrated." In this and other prominent first-generation ads, SKF emphasized pharmacological rationality, by implication associating thyroid hormones with harmful quackery.[58]

Starting around the beginning of 1951 and coinciding with a major new public health campaign against obesity launched by Metropolitan (see below) as well as psychiatric theories like Hamburger's, a new wave of heavy SKF advertising appeared in medical journals that pushed amphetamine's ability to help patients lose weight by treating their psychiatric problems. One of the earliest ads of this kind attacked the "popular misconception" of "the happy fat man." Under an image of a classical Chinese sculpture of a smiling man, the text explained that modern "physicians know that overweight not only takes years from life, but that it is usually the result of overeating—usually as the result of underlying depression." Benzedrine "curbs the fat man's appetite" to help him stick to his diet and "counteracts the mental depression" causing his habitual overeating. Similar ads from the early 1950s attacked traditional views, as represented by Chaucer's Wife of Bath and Friar Tuck of *Robin Hood*, that "fat people [are] . . . happy people." Instead, these ads claimed, fat people are "miserable"; they would benefit from amphetamine to "counteract the mental depression" driving their overeating.[59] By the mid-1950s, SKF's advertisements had fully embraced the psychiatric model of obesity, including overeating as a form of addiction. A full-page ad from 1955 entitled "Depression and Obesity Often Go Hand in Hand" told doctors that "you may find that the reason for [patients'] obesity is a depression that drives them to overeating—just as other patients may be driven to drinking."[60]

As the dominant amphetamine manufacturer among the major drug firms throughout the 1950s and 1960s, SKF spent heavily on advertising in medical journals to maintain that leadership. Its marketing campaigns reinforced the psychiatric understanding of obesity, especially the oral fixation theory, in the medical imagination. Some of SKF's competitors also produced ads for their own commercially successful weight-loss pills based on methamphetamine and (after the patent's expiration in 1951) amphetamine, which referred to mental ill health as an underlying cause for obesity, albeit never to the same degree as SKF.[61] But SKF was the only firm deeply invested in amphetamine's status as a psychiatric drug.

Both popular and medical understandings of obesity changed dramatically around 1940. Psychiatrists wrested control away from endocrinologists as researchers undermined the scientific evidence linking hormones and metabolism to obesity and developed new theories of overeating. They did so at just the moment that psychiatry was gaining status as a field in medicine and making itself central to American

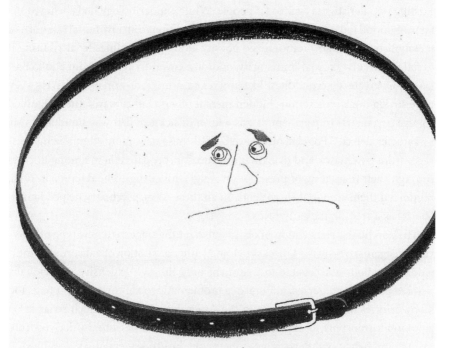

Advertisement for amphetamine diet pills that drew explicitly on the psychiatric theory of oral fixation. Source: *Journal of the American Medical Association* 159, no. 18 (1955): n.p.

national security and happiness. Further promoting the shift, the new theories of obesity as a reflection of a frustrated, immature self closely aligned with the pre-existing popular stigma against fat people. While endocrinology had sheltered the fat from moral judgment by attributing their condition to an involuntary abnormal metabolism, psychiatry remoralized obesity along popular lines by attributing it to failed initiative, sexual immaturity, and/or a cowardly retreat from adult challenges. Overeaters were addicts, like junkies or drunkards—or, alternatively, they were struggling with a serious hidden mental illness. Either way, fatness signified a grave psychiatric impairment; it was a form of sickness that was simultaneously a character defect.[62] Popular media welcomed these new, more stigmatizing messages from psychiatry, and drug manufacturers propagated them among doctors through their marketing of prescription weight-loss drugs. The doctors, in turn, reinforced them among their patients. In all these ways, psychiatry helped launch obesity as a crisis in the early 1950s.

The psychiatric reinvention of obesity also set the stage for a new type of intervention against obesity, as I discuss below. Neither a question of a disordered individual metabolism accessible to treatment only through expensive, individually tailored hormone therapies, nor one of a problematic social environment (e.g., too many calories or too much sugar in the American diet or too much reliance on automobile transport, all explanations suggested at the time), obesity derived from mental and behavioral flaws. Therefore, public health leaders quickly realized, it could potentially be addressed by altering individual decision-making through the type of intervention today known as "health promotion." In the increasingly conservative Cold War milieu, American public health practitioners trying to control heart disease found that such interventions, aimed at altering an individual's lifestyle (imagined as freely chosen), encountered far less resistance than many other approaches—particularly those impinging on the prerogatives of the nation's businessmen-physicians as represented by the AMA.

The sweeping success of obesity's psychiatric reconceptualization raises further historical questions about the early postwar cultural atmosphere of the United States, in which nonconformity or deviance excited an increased sense of threat as compared with the 1930s (e.g., high-profile campaigns to suppress drug addiction and juvenile delinquency and to root out hidden homosexuality and socialist sympathies).[63] As mental health advocates like Schlaifer made clear, Americans' new responsibilities as world leaders of the struggle against communism required a psychiatrically certified strength of character; this was a siege mentality posture in which the mentally unfit were but one step removed from traitors. The newly intensified, morally freighted stigma around fatness would be drawn on by public health as an instrument to alter individuals' behavior in a national campaign against the obesity epidemic, in the hopes that more would muster the willpower to lose weight in order to escape the combined social and physical penalties of fatness.[64]

CHAPTER 3

The Postwar Heart Alarm

In February 1948, the American Heart Association kicked off a major publicity campaign for the second annual National Heart Week with a supportive statement from President Truman (drafted by the AHA) that foreshadowed the role of health in the emerging Cold War: "America's first line of defense, the health of its citizens, is challenged by a formidable enemy which literally strikes a deadly blow at our national life." Truman's statement also included a phrase that would become increasingly familiar to Americans: "One out of every three deaths in the United States is caused by . . . cardiovascular disease." Heart-shaped plastic donation boxes captured coins on drugstore counters nationwide. A brochure entitled "One Out of Three" explained to people that donations to the AHA would help reduce this dreadful toll, and the message was spread locally through talks to civic and business groups. A radio campaign connected to the popular program *Truth or Consequences* brought in $1.8 million in donations.[1]

The National Heart Week campaign did not focus on obesity or any other likely causes of heart disease. It was mainly about raising funds to help the AHA conduct research to understand and eventually vanquish this scourge. While many epidemiologists believed that obesity—along with hypertension and a few other factors—lay behind the frightening national rates of heart disease, their opinions were based primarily on life insurance data and morbidity studies not specifically designed to address the question. Some were ready to launch public health interventions based on what was already known, but all agreed that they wanted more research into the causes of heart disease. So did the American public. Enjoying peace and prosperity for the first time in two decades, but shadowed by gathering clouds that foretold a new struggle with communism globally and possibly in their own midst, Americans turned inward to domesticity and personal fulfillment. In this context, the chronic diseases preventing a healthy, full life, including those associated with middle and older age, took on new importance as threats to what the nation held dear. According to a national poll that followed Heart Week in 1948, an astonishing 80 percent of the public wanted the government to spend hundreds of millions of dollars on research to fight heart disease, and they were willing to pay higher taxes for this purpose.[2]

In addition to the receptive context, new information helped raise the alarm. While heart disease had long been the leading killer nationally, in 1948 there was convincing new evidence that its dramatic increase since 1900 was not just due to lengthening lifespans. Death rates in the disease category had nearly doubled *after* accounting for age structure. And almost that entire increase was due specifically to rising coronary heart disease (CHD) deaths of people over the age of forty-five. "The majority of victims are robust, stout, professional[s] and businessmen"—the backbone of the economy—medical columnists explained. Soon, hard numbers supported the impression that the mounting threat was mainly to white males: their heart disease death rates in middle and older age groups were twice those of white females and had risen sharply since 1900, while rates among white females were declining. (Nonwhite men and women both showed higher heart disease death rates than their white counterparts, but for them too the trend was favorable or stable.)[3] Congress was so impressed with the public response to the Heart Week campaign of 1948 and the opinion poll—and, one may speculate, the white male death trend, which menaced politicians personally—that it passed the National Heart Act without much debate, creating the National Heart Institute and accelerating the growth of the National Institutes of Health. Soon, the NIH poured so many millions of dollars into heart research that the AHA's own burgeoning funds seemed trivial.[4]

In 1948, however, the new excitement around health and disease had to do with more than just research. For ambitious proponents of the new public health, the rising tide of morbidity and mortality from heart disease (and other chronic diseases) rationally demanded—and politically justified—massive new government involvement in health services. In early May 1948, with the Heart Act on its way to Truman's desk, the national Sunday newspaper supplement *Parade* carried a feature entitled "Wanted: Better Public Health" written, rather unusually, by a high federal official. In it Oscar Ewing, the new chief of the Federal Security Agency (the parent agency of Social Security, the Public Health Service, the NIH, and the Food and Drug Administration), described the ongoing work of the National Health Assembly, a commission he had convened to develop a ten-year plan for reforming the nation's health system. Ewing's piece opened by attacking Americans' complacent belief that they were "the healthiest nation in the world." Although public health had made good progress against maternal and infant mortality, typhoid, and tuberculosis, he warned that the United States ranked well behind other developed nations in combating these and other major causes of death. He reminded the public that during the war, 5 million draftees had been rejected as unfit to serve, and another 3 million were discharged for preexisting health reasons. About 25 million Americans were suffering from a serious chronic disease, accounting for at least a billion lost days of productivity annually. Heart disease alone accounted for at least a billion dollars of annual economic loss. The burden of ill health was staggering. And no wonder, argued Ewing, given the great shortage of doctors, dentists, nurses, and "organized public health services" in many parts of the country. Ewing, with the assembly's blessing, would solve these problems directly by having the federal government provide enhanced public health services and, controversially, medical care. But research too was important, Ewing said. In particular he thought that the research work of the National Cancer Institute, which accounted for more than half of the federal medical research budget, should be matched with proportional attention to heart disease (the most lethal disease) and mental illness (the most costly disease by many estimates). For Ewing, a supporter of the Heart Act, increased research funding should be yoked to a master government effort to expand and marry clinical medicine with public health nationally.[5]

Louis Dublin, a major architect and executive of Ewing's Health Assembly, had hoped that a "[broader] public health program for the country as a whole" finally would come from the assembly's efforts ("broader" was penciled in afterward in his letter to Metropolitan Life Insurance's president, implying that Dublin saw America's existing public health system as negligible). Soon, however, Dublin felt disappointed that Ewing replaced most of the public health experts he had recommended for the assembly with political allies and consumer representatives. Still, what emerged was essentially an updated version of the plans sketched at the National Health Conference a decade earlier, in which Dublin had also played a key role. These plans featured locally based health councils through which public health departments would coordinate comprehensive health services, including hospitals and physician care—funded federally through a national health insurance plan to be integrated into Social Security. With other new public health advocates, Dublin had long urged such coordination and an expansion of health insurance coverage to near-universality. The assembly's recommendations became a key plank in the Democratic campaign in the 1948 election, and afterward they were the basis for the Truman administration's health policy initiative—the Ewing Plan. The medical profession in 1948, with the *Journal of the American Medical Association* editor Morris Fishbein as its voice, recognized the same program of "socialized medicine" it had fiercely opposed a decade earlier and denounced the "emetic" of "compulsory sickness insurance." A monumental clash was coming, and what should be done about obesity and heart disease would hinge on the larger question of government's proper role in health.[6]

Awareness, Advocacy, and the Rise of the AHA

The dramatic elevation of heart disease in public consciousness coincided with a more general surge of enthusiasm for scientific research among the American public, which physicians too embraced. The scientific successes of the Second World War had catalyzed this new zeal. Not only had physics stunned the world with the atomic bombs that concluded the war, but the biomedical sciences had introduced penicillin, banishing a wide range of the most feared diseases (for example, venereal diseases and pneumonia) as matters of grave concern. The public embraced the idea that most illnesses could soon be conquered through intensive research. Earlier portents of this mood include the founding of the National Cancer Institute in 1937 and the phenomenal success of the National Foundation for Infantile Paralysis (NFIP), whose fundraising for polio research (as well as care and prevention) had by 1940 far outstripped that of all other voluntary health organizations.[7]

Inspired by the NFIP's success, the American Heart Association spent the war years reinventing itself. For nearly two decades from its founding in 1924, the AHA was dominated by academic heart specialists and by public health physicians specializing in rheumatic heart disease, a major killer that lent itself to public health approaches to prevention and control. Still, the budget and membership rolls remained small. During the late 1930s and the war years, however, the AHA's leadership shifted toward a younger generation of elite cardiologists oriented toward questions of physiology. Under this new leadership, the AHA established the professional certification exams that defined qualification in the specialty.[8]

The AHA's new, younger leaders envied the fundraising successes of the American Cancer Society, the National Tuberculosis Association, and the NFIP, which had brought visibility and resources to prominent academic centers and researchers in the sponsored medical fields. In 1942 the AHA hired the former publicity director of the National Tuberculosis Association as a consultant to assess its own potential to expand activities in a similar way. The consultant's report was encouraging: the American public was eager to fight heart disease and would respond well to a large-scale fundraising campaign. But among the AHA leaders, there remained misgivings about whether the organization would be promising too much in committing itself to reducing the toll of heart disease directly. They proceeded cautiously, in search of a flagship project to raise the AHA's profile, attract philanthropy or other new support, and make a visible impact on the nation's health. Research would be funded alongside and as part of that flagship intervention.[9]

In 1943 Harold M. "Jack" Marvin, chair of the AHA's executive committee, began seeking outside advice from leading figures in public health. One of his early interviewees was David Rutstein, deputy health commissioner of New York City and recent chief of the Heart Disease Division in New York state's health department. In Rutstein's opinion, the AHA's greatest opportunity lay in combating rheumatic fever—his specialty. This dreaded condition, the most common cause of death in school-age children, begins with a typically mild streptococcal throat infection. When not fatal, the disease often leads to permanent heart damage—rheumatic heart disease—through a largely mysterious process involving the body's immune reaction. (Rheumatic fever, a huge problem in schools, was also an important problem on military bases during the war.) Rutstein recommended physician education programs to improve the disease's recognition, especially its cardiac complications. He also endorsed a controlled study to determine whether hospitalization improved long-term outcomes—compared with home convalescence alone—for children suffering from rheumatic fever. As a supporter of the social medicine approach, Rutstein also advised that all aspects of rheumatic disease control should be centrally managed and "integrated" within communities in order to reduce any overlap and duplication of efforts from the multiple health agencies concerned.[10]

Marvin consulted with other leading lights in public health, including the former New York City health commissioner Haven Emerson and the retired head of the Yale School of Public Health, C.-E. A. Winslow, the foremost proponent of the new public health (see chapter 1). Emerson cautiously agreed that the best opportunity for public health interventions probably lay in rheumatic heart disease, both because its infectious origins were better understood and because lowering its long-term impacts on the heart seemed a tractable research problem. Not nearly enough was known about hypertension and coronary disease, he opined. Much less cautious, Winslow declared to Marvin that public health's domain included "anything and everything which affects the health of human beings." Thus health officers should be just as concerned about heart disease and cancer as about traditional problems like typhoid-contaminated food. He distinguished between "optimists and pessimists" in both the traditional and new approaches to public health. The pessimists demanded "proof upon proof" before launching any preventive inter-

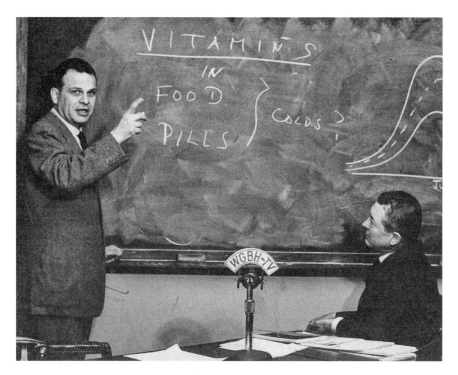

Preventive medicine professor David Rutstein of Harvard University, 1950s. Source: Francis A. Countway Library of Medicine, Harvard University, courtesy of WGBH Television, Boston.

ventions, but the "optimistic group," of which he considered himself a member, was "willing and anxious to try preventive methods, even without proof that they will be successful." From Winslow's perspective, the time was ripe for preventive campaigns against not just rheumatic heart disease but also hypertension and coronary disease—and the AHA had the responsibility to lead them.[11]

Thus encouraged, the AHA's leaders decided to enter the public health domain with a major program to fight rheumatic heart disease, on the grounds that the knowledge base was adequate and the time ripe. Their hand was in any case being forced by popular enthusiasm and momentum, including efforts by the federal Children's Bureau to form a national rheumatic fever foundation. (From the AHA's perspective, the formation of such a voluntary agency without its own leadership would be disastrous.) In January 1944 the AHA organized a conference in New York to discuss what should be done about the disease and what sort of national organization might be established to promote research and public health interventions.

Participants included representatives from the PHS, the Children's Bureau, the army, the navy, the Veterans Administration, the American Public Health Association, the Rockefeller Institute, and several medical institutions as well as experts in rheumatic fever.[12]

An important outcome of the conference was the formation of the Council on Rheumatic Fever under AHA leadership to advance the study, prevention, and treatment of the condition and to seek large-scale funds for doing so. By May 1945 the American Council on Rheumatic Fever, as it was now called, was formally constituted with bylaws, delegates (including some from the government agencies mentioned above), and a temporary executive committee chaired by Rutstein (who was by now a member of the AHA executive committee). Though fundraising lagged, the council moved ahead with publicity and popular appeals, for example in a national radio address by AHA executive member and leading rheumatic disease authority T. Duckett Jones (sponsored by Lederle pharmaceuticals, very likely because penicillin was at the time showing promise against rheumatic fever).[13] The AHA was taking its first uncertain steps onto a larger stage.

The AHA's flagship rheumatic disease initiative reflected Rutstein's ideas, especially once he formally became the Council on Rheumatic Fever's director in 1946. Indeed Rutstein's plans for a rheumatic fever demonstration project concretely embodied the new public health ideology: establishing up-to-date diagnostic facilities and cardiology consultation services for communities and schools; educating all doctors so that private physicians could serve public health by identifying new cases; creating special care facilities to isolate patients and develop specific therapeutic regimens; providing prophylactic care and rehabilitation services for recovered rheumatics; and so on, with programs benefiting rich and poor alike. He additionally proposed a registry, based on successful models from tuberculosis control, to which doctors would report all rheumatic cases. The registry would enable the health department to make sure that every patient received every health service she needed, whether through public or private providers, and also would allow researchers to follow up and track outcomes to see which interventions worked. The vision was of a rheumatic fever campaign on a "total community basis"—blurring the old lines between health care and public health campaigns based on contagion and also between research and clinical services.[14]

The plans Rutstein soon would propose for attacking obesity and the other factors associated with CHD would embody the same expansive vision. Another ambitious idea that the AHA hoped to fund was a large epidemiological study of the factors predisposing people to the main forms of heart disease, including coronary disease. This prospective study appears to have been conceived by the outgoing AHA president, Harvard cardiologist Paul Dudley White, as a "large . . . several year program to collect information . . . from entire communities" to measure the incidence of the major forms of heart disease "in relation to climate and mode of life." (By "mode of life" White primarily meant diet and occupation.) For the moment, however, it seemed out of reach for lack of funds.[15]

The AHA's leadership resisted the undignified "hullaballoo" required for a full-scale, national fundraising campaign to support either the rheumatic fever campaign or the proposed epidemiological study. In 1946, however, the organization did take steps recommended by its public relations consultant to transform the AHA into an NFIP-style super-charity by approaching eminent and wealthy people to join a "finance committee" for fundraising. The next year, the AHA launched a fundraising drive during the first-ever National Heart Week in February 1947. Slowly but surely, the AHA was becoming more ambitious.[16]

Dramatic changes in federal research policy overtook the AHA's slowly gestating campaigns. In the waning days of the war, Vannevar Bush, an MIT dean who had led one of the most visible wartime research agencies, had penned a long report (and soon after, a bestselling book) called *Science, the Endless Frontier*, which dramatized science's wartime contributions to national defense and health. With encouragement from the White House, Bush argued that the government should fund large-scale research indefinitely. This proposal was very well received and immediately taken up by congressional advocates of research.[17] However, differing visions divided the many lawmakers supporting the general idea of enhanced federal support for science—for example, differences over the degree to which the government should direct the science toward meeting national needs and differences about whether research funding should be distributed geographically to build capacity where it was lacking or instead be distributed according to the established excellence of researchers and institutions (inevitably favoring elite eastern universities). The convoluted political wrangling over the details of Bush's envisioned agency—which eventually became the National Science Foundation (NSF)—dragged on until 1950. In the meantime, the Public Health Service took advantage of the prevailing mood and the stalled genesis of the NSF by assimilating all the remaining biomedical research contracts from Bush's wartime agency into the NIH in 1946–1947.[18]

The congressional debates over the fate of the NSF gave health research advocates an opportunity to raise awareness of their favorite issues and plans. In mid-1946, through the AHA's publicity agency, Senator Harley Kilgore called Rutstein to testify before his science committee on the importance of heart disease generally and in particular the AHA's need for more funds to carry out its rheumatic fever initiative. Over the next few years, Rutstein and Duckett Jones would testify numerous times before congressional science and health committees, describing how the AHA was improving the diagnosis and care of patients with rheumatic fever, educating physicians and the public about heart disease, and funding research into its causes. While they always emphasized the AHA's accomplishments, they urged that they could do much more with greater resources.[19]

And extra resources were in the offing. Rutstein and Duckett Jones were summoned to Washington in the spring of 1947 to help Surgeon General Thomas Parran, Senator Claude Pepper, and Congressman Jacob Javits draft a bill that would establish a national institute for heart disease within the NIH.[20] With the help of a newly hired public relations counsel, Win Nathanson, they also prepared the kind of maximum-visibility fundraising campaign that had frightened them two years before.[21] As I discuss below, Rutstein would soon receive federal support to go ahead independently with some of the public health research and intervention plans that he had been hatching for years.

The National Heart Act was passed by Congress and signed into law by Truman in June 1948. The act established the National Heart Institute, which fell under the NIH's expanding biomedical research umbrella. By 1950, in addition to the National Heart Institute and the National Cancer Institute, the NIH included the National Microbiological Institute and the National Institutes of Dental and Craniofacial Research, of Mental Health, and of Arthritis and Metabolic Diseases. All six offered generous extramural funding to university researchers as well as labs at a growing Bethesda campus. From 1946 to 1950, the NIH annual budget ballooned from a modest $3 million to an unheard-of $53 million. Thus, before the NSF had even been created, the NIH had already become the chief patron of life sciences in the United States and indeed the world—and so it remained for the rest of the twentieth century.[22]

The 1948 National Heart Act displayed all the same ambiguities, conflicts, and mixed motives of the greater postwar biomedical expansion that spawned it. Its express purpose was to "improve the health of the people of the United States through the conduct of research" into the causes of heart disease, improve physician training, provide specialized diagnostic and treatment facilities for heart diseases, and support the "development of community programs for control of these diseases." This last mission overlapped the new public health expansionism reflected in the controversial Ewing Plan, entailing efforts to reduce the burden of heart disease in the present. The Heart Act also indirectly funded American medical schools through fellowships for both researchers and clinicians training in heart disease and through teaching grants to medical schools. Similarly, its provisions for laboratory-based research naturally benefited scientists working in medical schools and research hospitals as well as those at universities. In short, the Heart Act offered new money for projects favored across the political spectrum: enhanced government-funded public health care programs for those inclined to a greater federal role in health; arm's-length subsidies for teaching, advanced training, and modern hospital facilities for the doctors; and research funding to discover how to conquer—eventually—this leading killer of Americans.[23]

Cardiologists played a key role in shaping and administering these federal heart programs. The Heart Act required the surgeon general to create a National Advisory Heart Council (NAHC) to decide how the heart funds should be distributed via the National Heart Institute (NHI). This advisory council included several government officials from the PHS and the NIH, but representatives of medicine (mainly AHA officers) and the public (such as health research activist Mary Lasker) made up the bulk of the membership. Paul Dudley White was selected as chair, a choice that balanced well the triple demands of the moment—that government support science, the practice of cardiovascular medicine, and the public health. Effectively the dean of American cardiology, White had enormous credibility with both clinicians and researchers, having taught many of the nation's heart specialists directly at Massachusetts General Hospital and indirectly through his influential textbook. But as a longtime member of the American Public Health Association and the AHA, he was also intimately involved with public health activities: Rutstein's rheumatic fever project, for example, was initiated during White's tenure as AHA president. White vigorously advocated for the NHI in league with Lasker's circle of science promoters, sometimes achieving funding levels double what had been requested by a parsimonious White House budget office. To give but one example, in 1950 Congress appropriated $10 million for the NHI instead of the $4 million requested by the Bureau of the Budget, thanks largely to White. And when President Dwight D. Eisenhower suffered a heart attack in 1955, White become a celebrity as his doctor, further enhancing his influence.[24]

Through his foundational role as the National Advisory Heart Council's chair, along with his informal influence over both cardiologists and the NHI, White organized American research into heart disease in the 1950s. He began by convening a series of meetings and planning conferences in 1949 that involved nearly all the influential clinicians and researchers in cardiovascular medicine and many from

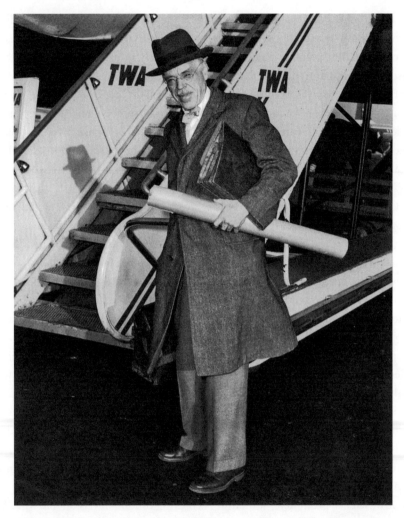

Harvard cardiology professor Paul Dudley White, 1950s. Source: Keystone Pictures
USA / Alamy Stock Photo.

public health and other domains. The eminences serving on the committees that
White created defined the cardiovascular disease situation and wrote the agenda
for research and disease control activity in the United States. The process culmi-
nated in the first National Conference on Cardiovascular Diseases, which was held
in Washington, DC, in January 1950 under the joint auspices of the AHA, the NHI,
and the NAHC.[25] While the greatest part of this planning activity was devoted to
cardiology training programs, surgical techniques, facilities, and the like, discus-

sions also dealt extensively with the major causes of heart disease—and what preventive medicine and public health could do to control it. Encouraging weight loss figured prominently as a key avenue for prevention, along with more ambitious public health measures.

Uncovering the Causes of Heart Disease

Among cardiovascular diseases in the mid-twentieth century, coronary heart disease ranked second as a cause of death (after the very general category "diseases of the myocardium," or weakened heart muscle, usually caused by other distinct heart diseases, including CHD). And despite suspicions that death certificate data reflected an increasing attribution of CHD as a cause at the expense of other conditions, its apparent rise was dramatic enough that few experts doubted that at least some recent increase was real. More controversial was whether there was an increase in CHD and other cardiovascular diseases over and above what could be explained simply by the population's lengthening lifespan together with the decline in other conditions that tended to kill people in their middle and later years (such as pneumonia). Some regarded both CHD and the related problem of hypertension as natural "degenerative" consequences of old age—nothing but a symptom of medicine's success. But as I noted above, the years 1948–1950 saw the release of strong new epidemiological findings from the PHS, albeit based on death certificate data, showing that the *age-specific* death rate for heart disease was rising sharply, particularly for white, middle-aged males, a rise driven by increasing CHD death rates. It seemed that CHD actually was becoming more prevalent and harmful.[26] In any case, heart experts agreed that CHD was the most common distinct killer and, since it was increasing, a paramount problem for their field.

A combination of pathological and statistical data indicated some sort of link between obesity and coronary heart disease. In CHD, the coronary arteries that feed the heart muscle become blocked, choking the blood supply and starving heart tissue to death. Even though most patients experience CHD as an acute event in the form of a myocardial infarction, or "heart attack," cardiologists and pathologists understood CHD to develop gradually through the process of atherosclerosis. Over time, deposits rich in cholesterol develop in arteries, and these fatty deposits develop further into fibrous tissue limiting flow through the affected artery and sometimes manifest in angina, a painful sense of chest constriction. When the narrowed coronary passages become catastrophically clogged, through a mechanism that remained uncertain throughout the period in question, a heart attack occurs.

While the root causes of atherosclerosis, its prevalence, and its epidemiology all stirred controversy in the 1940s, experts agreed that fatty deposits play a role. The idea that cholesterol in the blood contributes to cholesterol-rich deposits was widely entertained, although the straightforward suggestion that cholesterol in the diet lay behind dangerously high blood cholesterol levels fell into disfavor during the late 1940s. Evidence had emerged that the body itself makes most of the cholesterol in the blood. Whether obesity, a condition in which the fat content of the body is clearly excessive, contributes to atherosclerosis—either by raising blood cholesterol or in some other way—was another complicated question.[27]

To the insurance industry, the answer to many questions about the causes of heart disease were well enough known—not the detailed mechanisms of what happens in the body, to be sure, but the bodily signs and habits that reliably set odds on who would later die of heart disease. Louis Dublin's groundbreaking 1930 study had found that even men of moderately above-average weight for their height subsequently suffered elevated death rates from heart disease, diabetes, and stroke. In that study, Dublin classified overweight and normal weight in reference to the averages in his population. However, the men with the best longevity in that study were a little below average in weight for their height. And average weights crept higher still during the 1930s. During the war, Metropolitan issued new height-and-weight tables under Dublin's direction. The new tables defined an "ideal weight" for an adult man or woman of a given height, independent of age (but adjusted for slight, medium, or heavy frames, effectively broadening the limits). This actuarial ideal, or best, weight was simply that which predicted maximum life expectancy according to the latest data, and the ideal was well below the average weight (or median, the most common weight) for height in most age groups. That is, Americans were, as a population, now officially overweight, and their life expectancies were shorter because of it.[28]

An obvious implication was that Americans should lose weight to escape early death from CHD and other atherosclerotic diseases. The insurance industry was similarly certain about hypertension (high blood pressure). In addition to being a type of heart disease and a cause of death in its own right, hypertension predicted elevated rates of other cardiovascular causes of death, especially CHD and stroke. People with markedly high blood pressure, like those classed as obese, had serious trouble buying life insurance after the interwar period.[29] So, it followed, they should lower their blood pressure if they wanted to live longer (and merit lower premiums). In the late 1940s, how to accomplish that was not as clear-cut as how to reduce weight.

The insurance industry's epidemiology was good enough to enable companies to set premiums efficiently and to select insurance clients that in fact lived longer than average, but the evidence base did not give a full picture of the national population. Industry data came entirely from policyholders, who were whiter, wealthier, and healthier than the American population as a whole. For the scientific purpose of exploring the individual characteristics identified during medical examinations that predicted later heart disease, this was not a problem; the best lab rats for medical experimentation, after all, are more biologically uniform and free of extraneous illness than are natural populations. (In addition, from a political perspective, whiter and wealthier people were the citizens who mattered most.) But public health researchers wanted to know more about the prevalence of heart disease predictors, like obesity and hypertension, and the incidence and prevalence rates of heart diseases in representative samples of the actual national population. Furthermore, cardiologists and lab scientists studying heart disease were not satisfied with causes as inferred from epidemiological statistics at all. They wanted to understand CHD and other heart diseases in terms of the biological processes and mechanisms that gave rise to clinical manifestations, like heart attack, and to test theories about mechanisms through controlled experiments. When more knowledge of this type was gained by the scientists, they expected it would mesh with and help explain the epidemiological statistics and perhaps suggest new avenues for prevention and treatment.

At White's January 1950 national conference, leaders of the various research disciplines involved in heart disease were asked to assess what was known in their field to date and on that basis to determine what was most important to do and learn next about heart disease. In reference to atherosclerosis and CHD, separate panels of pathologists, cardiologists, and biochemists all essentially agreed that high levels of cholesterol (and other fats or lipids) in the blood serum probably contributed. They also agreed that the main questions that needed investigation were, first, what dietary and other lifestyle factors caused risky high serum cholesterol levels, and, second, why and how cholesterol in the blood became deposited in the artery linings. The panel discussing hypertensive heart disease, a related topic since atherosclerosis was thought to be a major cause and possibly also a result of hypertension, felt that its root causes remained a mystery; they wondered whether perhaps the nervous system or hormones were responsible for narrowing peripheral vessels, producing resistance to blood flow. However, that panel identified more potential interventions to retard the condition's development than had the atherosclerosis experts. These included a reduced-salt diet, weight loss, "physical and mental rest," the cultivation of serenity, and in some severe cases an operation to cut certain nerves.[30]

The reference to "mental rest" referred to a third major possible cause of the menacing rise in CHD, which also received considerable attention at White's national conference: emotional or occupational stress. There was some evidence that mental stress could produce relevant physiological reactions, including hypertension and perhaps even elevated cholesterol, and that evidence seemed all the more plausible because psychosomatic medicine was enjoying a degree of heightened influence. Behind the scenes, however, infighting between psychiatrists favoring and opposing the rising influence of psychoanalysis undermined the prospects for heart disease research in this field. White himself, probably representing many cardiologists, was downgrading his own estimation of the importance of the psychiatric factor at the time. Still, the idea that emotional strain could cause CHD retained its appeal among at least a fraction of American cardiologists, receiving some clinical and epidemiological attention in the 1950s and later enjoying a second life in the form of the Type A coronary-prone personality, a concept developed in the 1960s and 1970s.[31]

As for the public health researchers involved in White's national conference, they participated in panels assigned to the problem of assessing the actual prevalence of heart diseases in the population, the problem of which interventions could prevent or reduce the national impact of heart disease, and the more abstract epidemiological problem of measuring the importance of particular physical, nutritional, genetic, and environmental factors thought to contribute to heart disease (prominent among these suspected causes, of course, were blood pressure, obesity, mental stress, and serum cholesterol along with its dietary basis). This last research-oriented panel called for new, hypothesis-driven population surveys, especially prospective studies on representative population samples that would examine people at study entry and then again after a specific period, tracking deaths and major medical incidents along the way. This approach would allow measurement of the rate of new heart disease (i.e., incidence) and identification of the type of people who developed it, much like the insurance studies.[32]

The group concerned with assessing current prevalence agreed that they wanted studies of representative communities, both prospective studies in which a particular sample was followed over time to determine incidence rates, and cross-sectional surveys of heart disease morbidity to look at prevalence. However, while they agreed that much more needed to be known for ideal public health interventions, in the spirit of Winslow's "optimists" this panel believed that enough was already known to take significant action. For interventions to control coronary disease, as for rheumatic fever and other important forms of heart disease, they endorsed aggressive "case finding" coupled with mass screening programs that would capture large swaths of the population; they especially advocated for modifying tuberculosis screening programs using chest X-rays so that heart disease could also be identified (about which, see below).[33]

The committee concerned with prevention echoed that activist spirit, proposing to prevent heart disease with programs to educate the public about "weight control, body build, heredity, stress of modern living, smoking, drinking"—reflecting the list of major suspects behind CHD and hypertension (other than a "rich" diet), which by this time included cigarettes. The conference's central scientific and clinical expert panel also offered weight reduction as its chief recommendation for a primary prevention program aimed at CHD.[34] This last recommendation essentially endorsed an existing obesity control program aimed at reducing heart disease, which had already been under way for nearly two years. So too did the recommendations for mass screening and for a longitudinal study of heart disease in an entire community to look especially at CHD causes.

From Framingham to Screening and Obesity Control

While discussions of a heart bill were under way in Washington during 1947, Congress made a special $500,000 appropriation to the Public Health Service for heart disease work, and beginning from at least August 1947 public health researchers forged ahead thanks to this support. That month, a group of upper-level PHS officials met with Rutstein and Duckett Jones, representing the AHA, in the surgeon general's office to discuss what to do with the windfall. Joseph Mountin, the PHS's chief epidemiologist at the time, made a pitch for an "epidemiological field study on the incidence of cardiovascular disease," which was being planned by his subordinate Gilcin Meadors, to examine and then follow a population for fifteen or twenty years. Rutstein expressed great interest in locating the study in a town near Boston, where he would soon assume a Harvard professorship, and there was no sign of dissent. This plan would eventually become the Framingham study, which is foundational for our current understanding of the degrees to which factors like hypertension, smoking, and obesity contribute to CHD.[35]

However, in its original conception Framingham was not just a quantitative observational study. Mass screening was a long-term goal of Mountin and Meadors's initial plan in 1947, and group obesity control would soon emerge from a closely related pilot study. A draft plan dating from this time, likely the original Mountin-Meadors PHS proposal, calls for a nationally representative—that is, white and not recently immigrated—town of 20,000 people as the sample population, in which at least 12,000 people between thirty and sixty years old would be carefully examined and then followed up with repeat examinations after five years. Public health nurses would make contact with the participants at least annually between examinations to record new medical histories. The initial examination would include a detailed family and medical history; an assessment of features, including height, weight, blood pressure, and mental tension; several urine and blood tests, including serum cholesterol; and a number of "objective" physical measures of cardiovascular function by technicians. These objective examination techniques—for example, simplified electrocardiography, chest X-rays, and the use of a new instrument called the electrokymograph—were being tested as detectors and predictors of heart disease for their utility in future mass screening. In September 1947, with PHS encouragement, Rutstein and his friend Vlado Getting, the health commissioner of Massachusetts, were already planning for this prospective study focusing on hypertension and coronary heart disease to take place in Framingham. Bert Boone, Meadors's immediate PHS superior and the initial head of the Framingham project, was the electrokymograph's inventor, indicating the importance of mass screening in the Framingham study's original agenda.[36]

An idea at the very forefront of public health in the late 1940s, mass multiple screening was an intervention steeped in the new public health ideology and linked to the Truman health reform agenda of government-funded care managed by public health professionals. Mass screening had grown from wartime campaigns that used mobile X-ray units to identify and treat new cases of tuberculosis in entire industrial facilities or communities. What made the screening "multiple" was the simultaneous testing for other conditions; for example, in 1949 Lester Breslow, the California health department's chronic disease head, conducted a pilot project that took chest X-rays, blood samples, and urine samples from nearly 1,000 volunteers in four industrial plants near San Jose, examining all for signs of lung disease, heart disease, kidney disease, diabetes, and syphilis. Those testing positive were referred to physicians for confirmatory diagnoses, uncovering up to 30 new patients per 1,000 who would benefit from treatment.[37] But the mass screening concept had earlier roots in the town of Framingham itself. From 1916 to 1923 that community had hosted a successful disease control experiment, jointly created by the National Tuberculosis Association and Metropolitan Life Insurance. Its goal had been "to discover all cases of tuberculosis in the community, to determine the economic and social factors in disease causation with special reference to tuberculosis, to apply the best known methods of treatment, to develop a comprehensive programme of prevention, and organise the community for disease prevention and health creation." Young Louis Dublin, in his early position in Metropolitan's activist Welfare Division, played a leading role in designing it as a test of the new public health principle that putting local health officers—both lay and professional—in charge of a broad program of prevention, education, and medical treatment (including physician consultation and public clinics) could yield concrete dividends. And it did, halving TB death rates in Framingham compared with control towns by 1924. In choosing Framingham for the PHS project, Rutstein and Getting were likely imagining a similar program to remake health care systems on a city scale, treating the heart disease epidemiological study as a "community diagnosis" (as the Metropolitan investigators considered their TB initiative) whose chief purpose was not scientific hypothesis testing about disease causes, but formulating a guide to immediate prevention and control efforts—a comprehensive community treatment.[38]

Although a combined epidemiological survey and disease control intervention in Framingham suited Rutstein, by the end of 1947 the PHS separated these into distinct projects: a heart disease control program led by Lewis Robbins and an epidemiological study led by Meadors. While still reporting to Boone, the PHS Heart Disease Demonstration program chief based in Philadelphia, both were assigned to Massachusetts and located at Harvard formally under Getting's and Rutstein's authority (until they were transferred in mid-1949 to the NHI). The reasons for this separation are unclear; it may be, as historian Gerald Oppenheimer has argued, that the PHS wanted to protect the pure epidemiological research plan from Rutstein's interventionism—although Boone's job title indicates that for the PHS the epidemiology and heart disease control aspects were originally conjoined. Furthermore, in a letter to PHS superiors Meadors later blamed Rutstein for "alienating" the two aspects of the program, suggesting that the separation was unfortunate.[39]

Boone came to agree with Meadors and Robbins that "Dr. Rutstein should not be the basket in which all our eggs lie," and he, Mountin, and Estella Ford Warner, the head of state relations in the PHS, split the disease control demonstration from the Framingham epidemiology study and moved the former to another town yet to be designated. In early 1948 Meadors and his PHS team began fitting out examining rooms in Framingham and relocated there in mid-1948; free from Rutstein's micromanagement, they began to perform the initial examinations in that iconic study by the end of the year. As the study proceeded, the researchers quickly dropped diet and anxiety as risk factors under investigation, largely for practical reasons (they were hard to assess quickly and reliably), and focused on measuring what may be called the big three probable causes of CHD in late 1940s epidemiology: serum cholesterol, hypertension, and of course obesity. (Anxiety and some of the occupational or social class aspects of heart disease that interested Rutstein were reintroduced to the Framingham study in the 1960s.)[40]

Rutstein continued his active involvement in Robbins's heart disease control pilot study, which was relocated in mid-1948 to the affluent Boston suburb of Newton. By early 1949 this project too was under way, having received PHS funding as one of the earliest disease control projects supported under the Heart Act. What came to be known as the Newton Heart (or Heart Disease Control) Demonstration program can be viewed as a watered-down derivative of the Framingham TB pilot and another new public health showpiece of the 1920s, a cancer control pilot program conducted in Massachusetts. Like the Framingham TB program, this cancer pilot was overseen by the health department and undertook diagnosis and treatment at a community level. It involved both doctor and patient education, free diagnostic clinics, publicly funded outpatient treatment and hospitalization, and a registry of cases—both to ensure that all received help and to enable epidemiological investigation (of the characteristics of people most likely to have the disease and of their outcomes). Another key feature was oversight by a committee of local physicians in each community.[41]

The Chronic Disease Branch of the Massachusetts health department under Herbert Lombard, one of the 1920s cancer program's leaders, sketched an early plan for the Newton program under five headings, each led by a subcommittee that included local physicians: physician education, community organization (including education of the public), temporary voluntary reporting (i.e., a case registry), rehabilitation, and nutrition.[42] This last group initially concerned itself with the dietary needs of heart patients but was redirected to the problem of prevention through a spirited May 1949 address in Newton by Rutstein. He argued that based on insurance statistics, obesity was certain to contribute greatly to heart disease mortality, and he stressed the "psychological factor in obesity." Rutstein had obviously kept abreast of the latest psychiatric thinking on obesity, which linked the condition to alcoholism and other addictions. Conjuring a psychological solution suiting the mental problem of fatness, Rutstein proposed heart disease prevention through weight loss by using small therapeutic groups modeled on Alcoholics Anonymous, where "pride, vanity, fear, competition," and mutual support could assist overweight participants to stay on their diets.[43]

Rutstein's talk galvanized immediate action. Within a few weeks, a trial of a weight-loss intervention inspired partly by AA had been designed and launched. A dozen people referred by their physicians, all middle-aged and over their "ideal weights" by at least 15 percent but otherwise healthy, met weekly at the Newton YMCA for group discussions moderated by the program nutritionist; after six weekly sessions, another six followed fortnightly. There were guest lectures from health professionals on such topics as drugs and hormones in reducing, exercise, and mental health, but the emphasis was on sharing among peers. After six months, the group-discussion study was able to report that ten of twelve participants had lost weight, and five had reached their ideal weight. The participants, ten women and two men, called themselves "Gluttons Anonymous" and continued meeting for a time after the official sessions ended.[44]

An idea whose time was ripe, the Newton group therapy–weight loss pilot study excited enthusiasm among both clinicians and public health professionals. In late May 1949, even before it was actually under way, the Newton study's leaders already professed that its most promising opportunities in heart disease prevention were rheumatic fever control programs in schools, reducing bacterial endocarditis (a special problem for recovered rheumatics) through penicillin prophylaxis before dental procedures, and for CHD the "control of obesity." In obesity they saw a problem "almost as difficult as that of keeping an alcoholic sober," and given the profound "difficulties in achieving results by public health methods," the "techniques of Alcoholics Anonymous" were being applied to alter individual eating behavior. (Here, "public health methods" presumably meant population-level interventions, which were not impossible to imagine for obesity control; for instance, advertising controls on sweets and soft drinks modeled on alcohol regulation were proposed in 1942 by the surprisingly progressive AMA Council on Foods and Nutrition on the grounds that such sugary foods with low nutritional content cause widespread health harm.) In 1948–1949, in a review of public health approaches to heart disease control, weight reduction was the only preventive measure Rutstein endorsed for both essential hypertension and CHD.[45] The Newton study helped launch a massive national wave of group weight-loss studies and AA-inspired self-help fellowships, which I discuss below.

Doctoring the Masses

Mass multiple screening was sweeping American public health at the time—"one of the most attractive programs ever initiated by PHS," according to Surgeon

General Leonard Scheele in January 1950 although, he ominously added, "difficult to sell."[46] Indeed, the Newton demonstration also involved some mass screening for heart disease at a local factory. This last intervention was part of a much larger experiment in screening under way in Massachusetts at the time. The Massachusetts health department seems to have begun planning its multiple screening project in 1948 roughly simultaneously with Breslow's in California, within Lombard's Chronic Disease Division. As in Lombard's 1920s cancer control pilot study, he and Getting first won the Massachusetts medical society's approval to establish several public screening clinics that would test for heart disease, diabetes, and some forms of cancer; individuals with positive screening tests were referred to hospitals or private physicians. In 1949, with funding from the American Cancer Society, the AHA, the state medical society, and later the PHS, these clinics opened and continued operating into 1952—over time speeding and simplifying the tests so as to eliminate an examining physician entirely in favor of technicians and nurses. The final version involved a self-completed medical history; height, weight, hearing, and vision tests; simple blood and urine tests; fecal occult blood and Pap tests for cancer; and for cardiovascular disease a blood pressure test, a simplified (one-lead) electrocardiogram, and a chest X-ray (examined off-site for both lung and heart abnormalities). As implemented, it cost about $8 per person screened, but the Massachusetts team reckoned that the price could be brought as low as $2 with refinements.[47]

Rutstein participated in the Massachusetts multiple screening pilot project, researching methods for dealing more effectively with heart disease. He formally evaluated the dual use of a certain type of X-ray film used for tuberculosis screening, finding that the reading of the same chest films for both abnormal heart and lung shadows, followed by a confirmatory cardiological examination, discovered significant numbers of unsuspected heart disease cases in the course of a typical community TB survey. He also found that regular PHS medical officers had roughly the same confirmation rate (69 percent) as specialist radiologists (61 percent), so that a second set of film readers was unnecessary. To Rutstein, the discovery of 280 new patients with heart disease—about half of whom he thought would benefit from the diagnosis by, for example, going on a low salt diet to reduce blood pressure—in 31,000 chest X-rays was a powerful argument for heart disease screening in broader multiple screening programs.[48] Multiple screening fit well with the new public health concept, infused throughout Rutstein's planned rheumatic fever initiative, of an integrated program where the local health department would coordinate prevention, case detection, and clinical services. But who would attend to all the newly discovered heart disease patients so as to extend their lives—and save

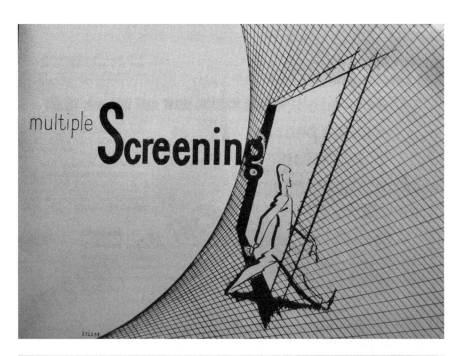

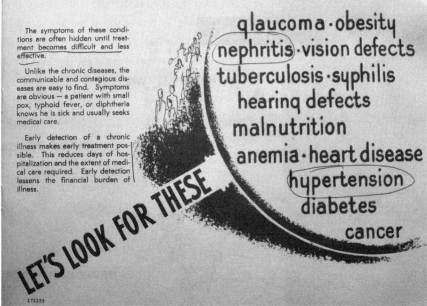

Public Health Service pub. 7, GPO 89-171155 [ca. 1950–1951], cover and internal page. Note how detection implies provision of medical care. The handwritten markings may be Rutstein's. Source: Francis A. Countway Library of Medicine, Harvard University.

taxpayer money? The experts at White's January 1950 national conference endorsed mass screening but noted that "there is limited value in case finding" unless afford-able care and facilities are available to all in whom heart disease is discovered.[49]

And this, precisely, was the political problem with mass screening, given the context of Truman's national health insurance initiative of 1949–1950 and the fierce physician resistance it aroused. Provision of care to all new cases was essential for the public to benefit from mass screening, so mass multiple screening in a sense pre-supposed and created demand for something like the Ewing Plan's near-universal health insurance. Aware or not of this implication, public health officials found mass multiple screening hard to resist. Along with Newton, two more of the six heart disease control research projects funded in the Heart Act's first fiscal year (1948–1949)—in Salisbury, Maryland, and Charleston, South Carolina—featured mass screening programs.[50] The next year (1949–1950), increased Heart Act dis-ease control funding saw multiple screening projects proliferate, including in Indi-ana, Virginia, Georgia, Alabama, and California.[51] A. L. Chapman, head of the new Chronic Disease Division within the PHS Bureau of State Services, urged in a 1949 article that multiple screening was good for the nation's people, who would stay well and productive as a result of early disease detection, good for taxpayers by reducing society's disease burden, good for public health officers, who would not only make progress against chronic illness but do so with a "tangible" service more easily appreciated by the public than milk inspection and clean water—and good for doctors, who would win fresh business.[52] Breslow too offered this conciliatory logic by insisting that screening results increased private physician appointments and even induced "many persons, who would perhaps otherwise not do so, to se-lect a personal physician." Breslow learned, however, that private practitioners still resented these screening tests as weakening the doctor-patient relationship (per-haps because they revealed diseases the doctor had failed to notice) and still feared them as the forerunner to "state medicine" (perhaps because the new cases created a demand for medical care far exceeding what private physicians could meet). As Lombard and Getting lamented, many "physicians . . . fear the program as the foot in the open door of state medicine," yet they hoped that doctors would come around because of the public health benefits and the new patients they would acquire.[53]

By and large, they hoped in vain. While mass screening and other heart disease control programs were proliferating with Heart Act encouragement in 1949 and 1950, fierce battles were raging over the Truman health reform initiative. Ewing's plan had many facets, but the flash point for controversy was the Social Security–

like provision that all employed people would pay a 1.5 percent tax, matched by their employer, to a federal agency that would fund insurance coverage for health care. Believing that this federal insurer would be in a position to dictate what clinical services were covered and at what rates, the AMA savagely attacked the plan, outspending its adversaries nearly fifteenfold with what can only be described as a lavish fearmongering campaign. One example conveying the flavor of the AMA publicity offensive is a pamphlet falsely describing the 1.5 percent tax as "from 3% to 10%" of income. Another "question" addressed in the same pamphlet was "Would socialized medicine lead to socialization of other phases of American life?" "Lenin thought so," the pamphlet answered. "He declared 'socialized medicine is the key-stone to the arch of the socialist state.'" Some senators eventually obtained a letter from the Library of Congress stating that there was no record of such a statement in Lenin's speeches or writings. That is, the AMA's publicity agency fabricated it, but it effectively forged an imagined link between health insurance and the advance of communism in the first fearful days of the Cold War. The AMA's lobbyists continued to maneuver behind the scenes to prevent passage of any administration-backed health care bill before the midterm federal election of 1950.[54]

By the end of 1950 the bold and optimistic spirit with which the postwar American public health community had approached heart disease control, especially mass screening, had ebbed. That spirit had been on show in late 1948, when an elite steering subcommittee for White's national conference endorsed the principle that heart disease control grants to states should contribute to "complete health programs for individual and community"—very much in tune with the new public health and Truman's health initiative.[55] The heart disease control activities actually undertaken by health departments with PHS support were more modest, commonly involving heart disease awareness publicity, screening with physician referral for confirmation, rheumatic disease initiatives in schools, and (increasingly) group weight loss. But it did not take long for even these halting efforts at expanding the role of public health to provoke strong resistance—which nobody knew better than Paul Dudley White, who was seated at the intersection of cardiology and public health as the NAHC chair.

The greatest conflict emerged around case finding, particularly in the general population via mass screening. Rutstein sensed trouble in August 1950, worrying that certain unproven screening procedures promoted by Chapman's Chronic Disease Division would discredit the whole multiple screening concept—and open the PHS to further "attack by the organized medical profession."[56] By October 1950 Rutstein's fears came true when, in White's view, tensions around screening grew "threatening and sometimes explod[ed] in several places, in particular in Illinois, Texas, and Hawaii," and probably elsewhere too. Rebuking the PHS and NAHC members involved with heart disease control (including Chapman and Rutstein), White described private physicians' mounting antagonism and "fear . . . of invasion of their own privileges, rights, and opportunities." He sympathized with the doctors "when, for example, it is proposed to establish diagnostic clinics where there are already excellent private clinics" with which a public clinic might compete. Public diagnostic clinics only "should be established *with the approval of the local medical profession*," White's memo practically shouted. Further, White blasted the "current fetish" of newer screening techniques, "such as ballistocardiography or fluorokymography or electrokymography or mass X-ray detection of tuberculosis or even cardiac catheterization"—all of which he regarded as experimental or suitable only for hospital use. Rutstein must have been dismayed to see White lump his chest X-rays together with "fetishes," for which Rutstein blamed Chapman. White concluded by admonishing that "we *must correct* the situation," and an essential starting point would be to require that a "widely recognized and respected expert" in cardiovascular medicine "and not an administrative health officer alone" have responsibility for each state heart disease control program.[57]

White's last suggestion was quickly put into effect, making oversight by the local AHA branch a universal feature of state heart disease control programs and thus subordinating public health to the clinical specialty of cardiology.[58] One reason for acquiescence by the PHS can be found in the November 1950 federal election, just a month after White sounded the alarm around screening. The American Medical Association had worked closely with the Republican Party to make fear of the Ewing Plan—"socialized medicine"—a winning "single issue aggressively sold to the voters" (as a Republican National Committee report put it). The propaganda barrage was intense and extended beyond standard advertising. Doctors wrote their patients individually using form letters provided by the Republicans and, along with dentists and nurses, campaigned door-to-door. While Democrats held on to slim majorities in both houses of Congress, few politicians afterward were willing to risk their careers for health reform. National health insurance was now a "dead duck," as the *Washington Post* declared in its post-election analysis.[59]

But the impact was far broader. As Truman lamented in 1951 to his confidante on health matters, Mary Lasker, Congress had turned "against almost anything

> ## CAN YOU ENJOY YOURSELF UNDER A FORCED STATE OF
> # SOCIALIZED MEDICINE?
>
> **DO YOU WISH YOUR CHILDREN TO GROW UP UNDER SUCH A STATE RATHER THAN IN A FREE AMERICA?**
>
> On Saturday, October 22nd, Ex-Governor Lehman released a letter from President Truman in which the President stated "the New York Senatorial race is being watched from coast to coast."
>
> This can mean only one thing. If Ex-Governor Lehman is elected it will be a go-ahead signal for President Truman to push socialized medicine on this country.
>
> **THE RECORDS OF THE TWO MEN PLAINLY STATE THEIR STAND ON THIS IMPORTANT QUESTION!**
>
> **MR. HERBERT H. LEHMAN — DEMOCRATIC CANDIDATE**
>
> Mr. Herbert H. Lehman, Democratic candidate for United States Senator in his opening campaign address September 22nd, 1949, pledged himself if elected to help carry out the Truman Fair Deal Program. "Socialized Medicine" is an important part of that program.
>
> "I am very much in sympathy with the principle of health insurance—it is my belief that it should become a part of the Federal Social Security Program."—*Herbert H. Lehman, Annual Message to the State Legislature, Jan. 3, 1940.*
>
> **SEN. JOHN FOSTER DULLES — REPUBLICAN CANDIDATE**
>
> Senator John Foster Dulles, the Republican candidate has taken a clear stand AGAINST Socialized Medicine. He is diametrically opposed to Mr. Lehman on this issue. Typical of his point of view are these remarks from an address at Elmira on September 19, 1949:
>
> "Socialized Medicine means regimentation of the finest body of Americans we have — dentists, physicians, surgeons, nurses — people who have worked loyally with devotion to their patients."
>
> ## "I have seen this scheme tried in Russia and England and I say to you it is utter catastrophe"
>
> ### Do Not Be Indifferent: Vote on Nov. 8th
> ### Protect the American Way of Life
> **Independent Group of Dentists and Physicians**

The Republican Party worked closely with the AMA and other doctors groups to make the Truman "socialized medicine" plan for health insurance a significant issue of 1949–1950 federal politics. Source: *Schenectady Gazette*, November 2, 1949, 13.

that has to do with public health." Multiple screening only flourished in those few "group practices" that, like Kaiser, developed into what became known as health maintenance organizations, with the resources and incentives to follow up on findings and (unlike private physicians) in a position to benefit financially from the strategy's long-term cost-effectiveness. America's public health leaders had to find ways forward that were more congenial to private practitioners than the coordinated system of publicly funded disease surveillance, preventive services, and clinical care that many had long sought.[60] For the optimists still intent on heart disease prevention, the cheap, individualist, and voluntary strategy of group weight loss for the obese became an obvious choice and the pathway of least resistance.

CHAPTER 4

Fighting Heart Disease One Calorie at a Time in Cold War Suburbia

The doom, for all practical purposes, of President Harry Truman's health reform at the end of 1950 presented a puzzle. Even if the American system of providing health care was the best in the world, as the American Medical Association liked to claim, the richest nation on earth was not all that healthy. And even if some Republicans opposed to federal involvement in health care, such as Senator Forrest Donnell of Missouri, disputed international comparisons by pointing out that *white* Americans enjoyed nearly as good a life expectancy as residents of nations at the top of the charts (Scandinavian countries and New Zealand), nobody could deny that heart disease, cancer, mental illness, and other chronic diseases were costing billions.[1] As the Cold War set in, the health of the free world's leader and self-proclaimed example to all other nations became something of an international embarrassment and a strategic liability. Heart disease was rising (at least among white males), Americans were too fat, and to many it seemed that something more than just research had to be done about this conspicuous threat to health and well-being. But that something could not be what the AMA called "socialized medicine."

While the federal expenditure on medical research continued its phenomenal growth in the early 1950s, federal support for public health activities declined steadily after 1951. Public health officials found no relief for their persistent "fiscal malnutrition," as one state's health commissioner put it in 1957.[2] In a context where the provision of large-scale, government-funded clinical services was off the table, the field's leaders had to reimagine health policy in the United States. To find a way forward and also to protect Democrats from another physicians-Republicans joint attack in the 1952 federal election, Truman appointed the Commission on the Health Needs of the Nation in early 1951 with surgeon and former Veterans Administration medical chief Paul Magnuson as its chair. For two years Magnuson's commission deliberated, met with panels of experts, and held open meetings around the country. The members enjoyed speeches like that of California Medical Association president Lewis Alesen, who denied any problem with American health care and decried all government involvement in it, based on the curious argument that "in Russia, under communism, the workman can buy one third quart of milk with his hour's labor," while in postwar England "under socialism . . . he can buy three," and "in America, under private enterprise" he can buy six quarts—and in addition, the United States had 94 percent of the world's televisions and 85 percent of all automobiles. The commission's findings generally supported the emerging trend of private health insurance subsidized by employers, which would help fulfill the hope that "everyone should have a personal physician."[3] The country needed more hospital beds, more outpatient services, and greater prevention efforts. And of course it needed to fund much more medical research, which was by now a bipartisan and uncontroversial view.

But, according to the commission, what the country needed most of all was for Americans to choose healthier behaviors. As a synopsis of its findings put it:

> The individual effort of an informed person will do more for his health and that of his family than all the things which can be done for them. In the past, measures for health and maintenance [e.g., sanitary water or milk inspections] demanded individual responsibility only to a limited degree. . . . Future accomplishments, however, depend to an even greater degree upon the individual's assumption of responsibility for his own health. It is the individual who must consult his physician for early care, avoid obesity and alcoholism, and drive his automobile safely. These things cannot be accomplished for him.[4]

Not coincidentally, this editorial only mentioned health threats that Americans could plausibly control on their own: obesity, substance abuse, and accidents. The way this foregrounding of "lifestyle choices" (as we now say) echoes the individualism and voluntarism that quickly became standard in American social sciences—and even required for political acceptability in the age of Joseph McCarthy—is obvious. So is the way this emphasis could help protect any intellectual field tainted with "socialism." Public health professionals henceforth should teach Americans how to help themselves, thus reaching an accommodation with clinical medicine at a historical moment when the latter enjoyed particular political clout and unprecedented public esteem (thanks to postwar wonder drugs and impressive new biomedical technologies).[5]

While this emphasis on voluntary and individual approaches to solving collective health problems was self-consciously acknowledged, the early 1950s marked a turning point that American public health leaders could not have foreseen: education, an established technique to modify public behavior (for example, teaching people to cover their mouths when coughing or how to safely dispose of waste, topics of many posters in the early twentieth century), would gradually expand into efforts to shape private behavior. The profession's direct efforts to alter the physical and social environment would diminish, and by the late twentieth century what is now called "health promotion" became the chief strategy of public health.[6] The way in which the field handled the obesity problem faced by the United States in the 1950s illustrates both how this happened and the problematic outcomes such a focus on individual behavioral choices can bring.

Group Therapy for Obesity

In the early 1950s, with mass screening stalled in the face of physicians' hostility and slumping budgets, American public health authorities embraced weight loss as an approach to heart disease control. Health departments could sponsor group weight-loss programs on the cheap, since they typically required only the publication of educational materials and the occasional services of a nutritionist, who was often on the health department staff already. Private physicians raised little resistance, since they often saw obese patients as uncooperative and undesirable clients. In any case, group therapy did not interfere with doctors' bottom lines, since the practice posed no obstacle to amphetamine (or thyroid) prescribing and involved no clinical services they otherwise offered. It might have bothered some psychiatrists, but as a specialty they were in short supply and high demand in the 1950s. Even the AMA endorsed group weight loss. Last but hardly least, not only did group-assisted weight loss fit the political tenor of public health in the 1950s, as the field narrowed its focus to finding solutions to social problems in individual behavior, but it also fit with broader cultural currents of the time, and the public eagerly embraced it.

The Newton Heart Demonstration may have hosted the first course of group therapy for obesity ever to be managed by health officials, but David Rutstein almost certainly did not conceive of the approach alone. In October 1949, only four months after the Newton experiment, the Public Health Service and the Massachusetts health department (whose chief, Vlado Getting, was in regular close contact with Rutstein) together began offering a pilot group weight-loss program through the Boston Dispensary. This larger and better-documented pilot study became at least as influential on subsequent programs as Newton.

Between the wars, the Boston Dispensary—then essentially a charitable community clinic—had housed a successful therapeutic group "class" on managing psychosomatic complaints, which was run by the tuberculosis specialist Joseph Hersey Pratt. The Pratt group meetings, also known as "thought control classes," have been described as an important forerunner of cognitive behavioral therapy in the United States. About twenty outpatients would gather around Pratt and, after some mental relaxation exercises led by him, would share their personal problems and their progress in turn. A session would conclude with sage exhortations by Pratt.[7] As the "class" concept indicates, special wisdom and healing powers were considered to reside in the charismatic medical expert leading the sessions, Pratt; the patients were not thought of as simply healing themselves.

By the mid-1940s, group therapy had moved in a more strictly confessional direction, with group members effectively learning from and helping heal one another, albeit under the paternal guidance of a psychiatrist or psychologist. The particular group therapy technique adopted in the Boston Dispensary study appears to have been developed by Benjamin Kotkov and other psychiatrists at the Veterans Administration hospital in Boston. During and immediately after the Second World War, group therapy spread among military psychiatrists as a timesaver to help them treat the many soldiers experiencing neurotic emotional disturbances (depression, anxiety, excess aggression)—what we might today call post-traumatic stress disorder.[8] According to Kotkov, the immediate goals of the group therapy technique were to diminish veterans' "feelings of uniqueness, stigma, and isolation"; promote their ability to accommodate "everyday reality" by strengthening their "group relationship and identification"; and loosen their "resistances" to adjustment based on "preconceived notions . . . on psychogenic problems." While participating veterans were asked to conduct a "self-inventory," the primary therapeutic effects were delivered through teamwork. This teamwork amounted to sharing anxieties, "unacceptable impulses," masturbation habits, and so forth with one another in search of an understanding that might help each person accept and manage his own demons. For Kotkov, the therapist in these sessions acted less as a leader than as a "permissive parental figure" and catalyst. The Freudian influence is obvious.[9]

Kotkov followed the general outline of his veterans program in developing the Boston Dispensary's weight-loss pilot program, although unlike the veterans, the participants in the study would not also receive individual psychotherapy. Working in collaboration with Stanley Kanter (a psychiatrist at Boston Psychopathic Hospital), PHS investigator Joseph Rosenthal, and nutritionist Marjorie Grant,

Kotkov used the group confessional format to uncover the underlying psychological conditions that drove the participants—mostly women—to overeat. Interpersonal encounters allowed each fat person to break down her terrible "loneliness," which was born of her sense of unique "unworthiness." They came to understand that their thoughts were no more "bad," "dirtier," or "inferior" than anyone else's. Gradually, participants shared their fears, hostilities, and lack of self-respect and explored the situations and urges making them overeat. Finally, through the airing and hearing of similar feelings and experiences, they each gained greater self-acceptance and a willingness to try eating less.

Although like the Newton participants they required physician approval, the Boston Dispensary's experimental subjects were not in the first instance referred by their doctors; rather, they were recruited through newspaper and radio announcements of a new weight-loss method—drawing far more responses than could be accommodated. After an initial evaluation, they were assigned to nine groups of fifteen to twenty each, which met for sixteen weekly sessions under a variety of discussion leaders or moderators. While all of the moderators could be described as experts on either health or human behavior, not all of them had a medical background. The facilitators included two teachers, a minister, a graduate student in psychology, two physicians, two psychologists, and two nutritionists. At the end of the four-month demonstration project, the investigators could say that, of those who finished the program, "the majority lost ten pounds or more." But there was a catch: only a minority of those who had enrolled initially completed the program. Those who did stick with it, however, found the program compelling enough that some chose to elect their own leaders and continue meeting regularly on their own. Among these devotees, the average weight loss one year from the start was an impressive 17 percent.[10]

Word of these two Massachusetts experiments spread widely among the public health community, stirring great enthusiasm. In Berkeley, California, researchers at the private Herrick Hospital launched a study in late 1950 in collaboration with Lester Breslow's Chronic Disease Branch of the state health department, which compared the psychologically oriented group therapy approach with a more traditional nutritionally oriented dieting class. Participants were recruited mainly by advertising, supplemented by a few physician referrals. So few men responded that the study soon limited the program to women and randomly assigned them either to the psychological therapy or the diet class groups. Each group included about a dozen women who met weekly for sixteen weeks under the guidance of a group leader with relevant professional expertise (in nutrition, psychology, social work, medicine, or public health nursing), closely mirroring the Boston Dispensary study's design.[11]

The Berkeley study produced encouraging—and intriguing—results: group weight loss worked, but there was no difference in effectiveness between the nutritional and psychological approaches. At the end of four months, four out of five participants who attended at least four sessions lost at least ten pounds. The investigators concluded that group discussion itself provided psychotherapeutic benefit without the need for mental health expertise. This study continued for two years, eventually accumulating usable results on 290 women, mostly around forty years old and married. While only about half of those enrolled lost significant weight (defined as ten pounds or more) in the sixteen-week period, as in Boston the success rate among those who faithfully attended was much higher.[12]

Another program, begun in late 1949 by diabetes specialist Joseph Goodman at the Cleveland Clinic, deliberately incorporated peer pressure into the therapeutic regime. In contrast to most of the other early group weight-loss programs embraced by physicians, Goodman and his collaborators do not seem to have drawn on any mental health expertise. Instead, small groups of overweight diabetics, mainly women, met weekly for a guided discussion that harnessed the participants' "camaraderie" and friendly competition. Each session began with a brief lecture related to obesity and weight loss after which the participants, whose weight charts were posted for all to see, subjected those who had not lost weight since the last meeting to "cross-examination." After meeting for nine months to a year, 90 percent of the Cleveland patients lost an average of fourteen pounds. The diabetologists thought that the group dynamic, particularly the fear of public shame, was the most important ingredient in their approach, even though the sessions were physician-led (considered essential for participants to feel accepted and supported).[13]

The Cleveland study was especially thorough: most investigators leading early group weight-loss studies declared success after less than six months. Skeptics quite reasonably asked whether the results would hold over time. Around the end of 1952, the Boston Dispensary researchers did a follow-up study to gauge the impact of the group approach after two years. They again claimed success: after two years, two-thirds of the group that had lost at least 10 percent of their excess weight had kept it off. Altogether, almost a third of those who stuck with the program for two or more sessions showed significant weight loss after two years. But even that modest claim was contested by a group led by Fred Stare, the head of the nutrition department in Harvard's School of Public Health. Stare pointed out that if the dropouts were included in the calculations, average weight loss was negligible by the end of the second year. In fact, he argued, participants lost the same amount of weight as the matched controls—overweight people who did nothing but receive a diet prescription.[14]

Stare, we now know, had a vested interest in discrediting weight-loss programs, which universally involved a "reducing diet" of 900 to 1,200 calories per day, emphasized lean meat and vegetables, limited fats and starches, and were hostile to calorie-dense sweet desserts (and almost any kind of snacking or treats). Through his research, popular articles, and congressional testimony, Stare consistently challenged advice and interventions that discouraged Americans from consuming sweetened foods, and he fought the implication that Americans' high sugar consumption was the cause of their obesity—as proposed, for instance, by Stare's colleague Joseph Aub when he taught Harvard's preventive medicine course during the 1950s. In appreciation for his help, Stare and his department were rewarded with generous funding (on the million-dollar scale) for research and facilities from the Sugar Research Foundation and processed food companies, such as General Foods. When Stare's extensive financial ties to the sugar industry finally came to light in 1976, he became the subject of scandal. In 1952, however, his attack on the Boston Dispensary study represented a reasonable critique of a public health intervention whose success was far from proven.[15]

But naysayers like Stare were the exception. At the time, weight-loss groups seemed to offer more hope for combating obesity—and therefore preventing heart disease—than any other tool available to public health professionals. In June 1952, the PHS's Chronic Disease and Tuberculosis Division convened a conference of researchers engaged with group weight loss (including representatives of the Boston, Cleveland, and Berkeley studies) to share experiences from their pilot studies and issue consensus recommendations to inform the spreading practice. All agreed on the centrality of addressing emotional problems when treating obesity. They recommended that groups of ten to twelve participants meet weekly for an hour for at least several months. They agreed too that the groups must always operate "under general medical guidance and close professional supervision" (leaving the way open for leadership by nonphysician professionals like psychologists, but not lay leadership). Opinion was divided over whether groups should be "closed" (that is, admitting only one cohort and lasting a finite period) or "open" (continuing indefinitely, with new members replacing lapsed members). The researchers thought the open format was better for "passive, dependent persons who need continuing support in their efforts to diet," but they thought the closed groups created greater "esprit de corps." From the presentations it was clear that far more women than men participated, but there was no sign of concern that as a result the approach might not actually impact heart disease (which was correlated more strongly with obesity in men).[16]

American public health professionals quickly embraced group therapy for weight loss as part of their fight against heart disease. By 1953, nineteen of fifty-four states and territories reported that they were conducting or planning such programs with PHS support.[17] Most of these programs explicitly followed the Boston Dispensary model, with expert moderators and roots in psychotherapy. As weight-loss groups gained in popularity, though, the public health community could not keep up with the demand. The group weight-loss movement soon evolved away from the PHS consensus that the practice required "medical guidance and close professional supervision."[18] Indeed, it outgrew the biomedical domain almost entirely.

America's Number One Health Problem

The PHS's interest in fighting obesity had emerged directly from its community heart disease control programs. As originally envisioned, weight-loss programs, screening for heart abnormalities, and preventing the spread of rheumatic fever were tactics in an ongoing war against heart disease. Within a remarkably short time, however, fighting obesity became an end in itself—for the American public if not for the PHS.

The insurance industry sounded the obesity alarm, obviously judging that the time was ripe. In mid-1951 Metropolitan Life launched an initiative, which had been planned for at least a year, to attack what it referred to as "Overweight: America's number one health problem." Louis Dublin and his colleagues announced the campaign in an address delivered at the AMA's annual meeting. Opening by pointing out that the nation's impressive progress in improving life expectancy had mainly benefited children and young adults, Dublin observed that little progress had been made against the chronic diseases afflicting the middle and later years, the United States compared poorly in this regard to many countries, and among middle-aged American men the death rates from these conditions were actually rising. Why? "Overweight is at the root of the high prevalence of the degenerative diseases in our country," he answered. Dublin reviewed the extensive evidence from the insurance industry and from smaller studies (on groups examined periodically, or based on autopsies), which showed that overweight and obese people suffered greatly elevated mortality rates from heart disease, especially from athero-

Metropolitan Life Insurance Company's 1942–1943 Tables of Actuarial "Ideal" (Best Life Expectancy) Weights

	Women (weight in pounds)				Men (weight in pounds)		
Height	Small frame	Medium frame	Large frame	Height	Small frame	Medium frame	Large frame
5'0"	105–113	112–120	119–129	5'2"	116–125	124–133	131–142
5'1"	107–115	114–122	121–131	5'3"	119–128	127–136	133–144
5'2"	110–118	117–125	124–135	5'4"	122–132	130–140	137–149
5'3"	113–121	120–128	127–138	5'5"	126–136	134–144	141–153
5'4"	116–125	124–132	131–142	5'6"	129–139	137–147	145–157
5'5"	119–128	127–135	133–145	5'7"	133–143	141–151	149–162
5'6"	123–132	130–140	138–150	5'8"	136–147	145–156	153–166
5'7"	126–136	134–144	142–154	5'9"	140–151	149–160	157–170
5'8"	129–139	137–147	145–158	5'10"	144–155	153–164	161–175
5'9"	133–143	141–151	149–162	5'11"	148–159	157–168	165–180
5'10"	136–147	145–155	152–166	6'0"	152–164	161–173	169–185
5'11"	139–150	148–158	155–169	6'1"	157–169	166–178	174–190
6'0"	141–153	151–163	160–174	6'2"	163–175	171–184	179–196
				6'3"	168–180	176–189	184–202

Sources: Metropolitan Life Insurance Company, "Ideal Weights for Women," *Statistical Bulletin of the Metropolitan Life Insurance Company*, October 1942, 6–8; Metropolitan Life Insurance Company, "Ideal Weights for Men," *Statistical Bulletin of the Metropolitan Life Insurance Company*, June 1942, 6–8. *Note:* Heights and weights are given with shoes and with indoor clothing on. These standards were propagated during Metropolitan's early 1950s campaign against obesity and overweight.

sclerosis and high blood pressure.[19] Heart disease appeared on Americans' death certificates, but the cause behind this cause of death was obesity (see table).

The Metropolitan researchers placed the national prevalence of overweight, defined as 10–19 percent above the actuarial best or "ideal" weight predicting the greatest life expectancy, at about 10 percent of the population (15 million of a total population around 150 million). An additional 5 million people were "seriously obese," a condition defined as 20 percent or more above ideal weight. Dublin and his colleagues acknowledged the uncertainty in these estimates, based as they were on unsystematic samples, but it seemed obvious to them that even a conservative estimate would condemn Americans on the whole as overweight.[20] Few expressed doubt about this prevalence at the time (though its importance stirred some debate).

Obesity might be lethal, but it was treatable. Metropolitan Life's campaign fully embraced the psychiatric model of obesity as a disease of overeating. Dublin and his colleagues warned the large audience of physicians that helping fat people, much as with alcoholics, demanded close attention to the patient's "personality, the social habits, the intelligence, the will-power, and capacity for self-discipline"— and of course the "emotional factors" behind overeating.[21]

In the same AMA meeting session, supporting Metropolitan, Northwestern University medical professor Clifford Barborka advised the physicians on prescribing weight-loss diets, warning them against unscientific fads and an overreliance on amphetamines. Amphetamines were dangerous, he cautioned, both because of their side effects and because they soon stopped working. A better solution was "group psychiatry" "classes," where difficult patients might share their "common problem . . . without fear of mockery" and eventually benefit from friendly competition and "mutual understanding and support." The obesity session was received with such enthusiasm among the doctors that the AMA repeated it in the December 1951 West Coast meeting with a "four day feature program urging physicians to take a firmer hand with overweight patients." At that meeting Dublin increased his national estimate of (combined) obesity and overweight prevalence from 20 million to 30 million, about 25 percent of the US adult population. Major newspapers carried the sensational story on the front page with headlines like "Unneeded Fat Hangs Heavy on ¼ of U.S."[22]

Metropolitan's campaign rested on surprisingly little evidence that losing weight actually improved the health of significantly overweight people—and the firm itself had generated what little they had. In 1950, Dublin and his colleagues had conducted yet another quasi-prospective study on Metropolitan's customers. This study examined the records of 50,000 men and women who were issued policies between 1925 and 1934, all of whom were initially charged extra because of overweight but were free of other "impairments." The group was followed either until their deaths or until 1950, and their mortality was compared to that of the insured population charged standard premiums in the same period. The policyholders who remained overweight were also compared to the subset who lost weight and sought lower premiums on that account. As expected from prior studies, Dublin found that excess mortality increased with the degree of overweight among both sexes; most of the excess deaths were attributable to cardiovascular and renal diseases and diabetes; and excess mortality among underweight people was becoming ever less significant (due to the retreat of tuberculosis). New and most important among their findings, though, was that overweight policyholders who lost enough weight to qualify for lower premiums also reduced their mortality nearly to what was expected in their new weight class. Thus, as Dublin put it, "fat people who lose weight live longer."[23]

There were problems with Dublin's study, as some skeptics noted. Rutstein, for example, felt that Metropolitan could not be sure that the overweight policyholders who were rerated after weight loss were the same in other ways as those who were not rerated. Rutstein argued that any person judged to be healthy by two medical examinations would live longer than otherwise similar people who only passed one, even if the time interval between the two examinations was corrected for—as Dublin had done. (This is because health problems undetected by the first exam might be picked up by the second.) Rutstein nevertheless granted that conclusive evidence could only come from an experiment that would probably never be done: randomly dividing an obese population into two similar groups, followed by the "reduction of one group to 'normal weight' and careful follow-up until all were dead."[24] And, indeed, that research has never been done. For quite some time, Dublin's study stood as the only direct evidence that losing weight could improve overall health, as measured by life expectancy.

Still, both doctors and the public health community were in general convinced; like the AMA, the PHS endorsed Metropolitan's national campaign against obesity. With timing and content that suggest deliberate coordination with the Metropolitan initiative, in 1951 the PHS published a brochure for public health departments titled "The Greatest Problem in Preventive Medicine in the USA Is OBESITY." The brochure reported the life insurance estimates of excess mortality from cardiovascular diseases, diabetes, and cancer, and it urged that people should avoid obesity to "stay healthy," "remain attractive," and "live and work more effectively." In keeping with the growing consensus, the brochure recommended that health departments sponsor weight-loss groups on the grounds that these help obese people manage the "emotional disturbances" behind overeating.[25]

Metropolitan developed a set of materials to convince the general public that overweight was dangerous and losing weight was desirable. A surviving relic is the firm's widely viewed 1951 educational cartoon *Cheers for Chubby*. The film tells the life story of a former high school athlete, Chubby Avoirdupois, who never adjusted his eating habits after his youth. On reaching middle age, Chubby begins to find his suits too tight. The film is distinctly harsher on the formerly "slim, attractive Mrs. Chubby," who has let herself go. She now has to buy dresses in the awning section of the department store—and on the way home, her derriere gets stuck in a taxicab door. When exercise and "fads" fail to slim them down, the couple go to see their

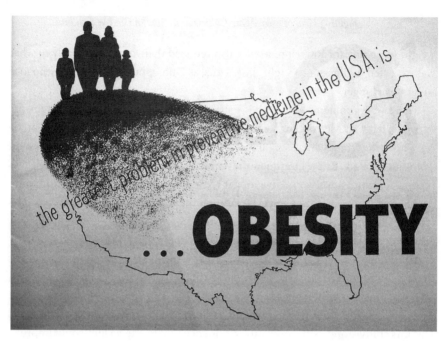

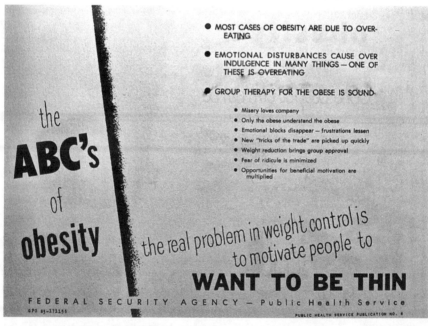

Front and back pages of Public Health Service pub. 6, GPO 171156 [ca. 1951], reinforcing the Metropolitan campaign against obesity. Source: Francis A. Countway Library of Medicine, Harvard University.

doctor. The helpful clinician explains nutritional basics and recommends a diet, advising them that "getting together with a group of other overweight people" would help them stick to it. Eventually, Mr. and Mrs. Chubby overcome the "devils" of tempting and hidden calories in foods like cake, pancakes with syrup, and butter, retrieving their good looks and vigor.[26]

So, in 1951 it seemed that all of the main parties agreed that the United States had a fat problem and needed to lose weight. The medical community and the pharmaceutical manufacturers that served them certainly concurred. The public health community was trying to propagate the group therapy approach for weight loss nationally, and the insurance industry was reaching out to both doctors and the general public with the message. People responded to the messages demonizing and, to some extent, further stigmatizing obesity, and many joined weight-loss groups. Soon the weight-loss groups took on a life of their own.

From Group Therapy to Overeaters Anonymous

When the soldiers came home after the Second World War, the young women who had been working in war industries left these jobs (voluntarily or not) and settled down to launch a baby boom—often in sprawling new suburbs far from the city centers where they had grown up and worked. Both men and women were isolated by this move, but it especially affected women, who were cut off from both workplaces and their extended families. While the young suburbanites turned inward to seek happiness in domesticity—comforts and conveniences for the home, a happy family life, and sexual fulfillment (within marriage) underwritten by the newly influential doctrines of Freudian psychiatry—they also had to invent new forms of sociability to counter the isolation. Husbands joined bowling clubs, teens went to drive-in restaurants and sock hops, and wives held Tupperware parties, joined the PTA, and organized local political campaigns.[27] They also joined weight-loss clubs. At first, most of these groups grew from or partnered with programs propagated by health departments. But over time, they diversified and outgrew the umbrella of medical authority, many of them drifting closer and closer to the spiritual self-help model epitomized by Alcoholics Anonymous (AA).

The Young Women's Christian Association played an important early role in spreading the practice of group weight loss along the lines encouraged by public health authorities. As the name suggests, the YWCA began as a philanthropic enterprise to save and uplift young women of the urban streets and working classes, but by the mid-twentieth century it was increasingly taking on a more middle-class and secular focus and rapidly establishing new branches in the expanding, leafy suburbs.[28] The Boston YWCA boasted a tradition of developing "cornerstone" programs, particularly in the area of health (introducing, for example, the first calisthenics program for girls), which the national association then rolled out to affiliates. It is unsurprising, then, that the Boston branch of the YWCA was the first to offer weight-loss groups, modeled on the Boston Dispensary pilot, in late 1950.

Although the Boston Dispensary researchers and the PHS indicated that the group leader or moderator need not be a health professional, the Boston YWCA's director of health services, Martha Gentry, deferred to medicine. Feeling it too risky to use a nutritionist because obesity essentially resulted from "emotional problems and not diets," she secured the services of psychiatrist Florence Swanson to lead the early groups. As Gentry and Swanson later described the program, the group meetings consisted of about fifteen women around a table for ninety minutes weekly for a total of fourteen weeks. The psychiatrist "didn't say much" (in the words of a participant), intervening only when necessary to keep the group discussion "on track." The group conversations stayed focused on food, eating, and "what was behind it all—why food was so important to us, what it was that seemed to drive us to eat as others are driven to drink." The answer lay in the participant discovering in herself an ingrained habit, retained from childhood, of seeking "satisfaction" through eating; this was in line with the oral fixation theory popular at the time. In classic psychoanalytic fashion, the individual insight gained through talk was itself the cure: "when we understood why we ate so much, eating wasn't so important anymore."[29]

The Boston YWCA continued this approach through 1956, subsidizing the cost of the psychiatrist for the modestly priced program and providing the compulsory consultation with a nutritionist—expenses that contributed to its ultimate discontinuation—and supplying materials and advice to other YWCAs interested in implementing similar groups. (The YMCA considered a similar program for men but never implemented it, maintaining its focus on sports.)[30] As historian Jessica Parr has related, these YWCA weight-loss programs achieved varying degrees of success. In mid-1952, for example, the inner Chicago (Loop) YWCA introduced a "group psychotherapy" program for obesity, drawing heavily on advice and materials from the Boston program. In collaboration with the PHS, University of Chicago psychologists, and the city health department, by 1953 the Chicago YWCA had established three types of therapeutic groups designed to test the Berkeley findings that the style and type of leader made no difference to weight loss (implying that the group itself was the therapeutic agent). In this particular case, the elaborate comparative research plan complicated the YWCA's ability to serve its clientele. The experiment seems never to have been completed, and after an initial burst of enthusiasm, the number of psychotherapeutic weight-loss groups offered by the Chicago YWCA dwindled. They ceased altogether in 1958.[31]

The experience of several YWCAs in Iowa was more straightforward and perhaps more typical. By 1953, the Iowa health department had established a heart disease control program featuring professional education in collaboration with the state's branch of the AHA, had plans for mass screening for heart disease in collaboration with the state's tuberculosis association, and had plans for obesity control. For the latter, the health department's Nutrition Division collaborated with the YWCA and other community organizations. The public health officials supplied instructional materials to anyone putting together a group as long as the organization had obtained approval from the county medical society and found a "qualified leader"—defined as a nurse, dietitian, doctor, or "home economics teacher who has special training in nutrition." By mid-1954, group weight-loss classes had been initiated in a dozen Iowa locations, of which half were run directly by the state health department, three by the YWCA, and three by other organizations. The group approach flourished, but by 1957 the state health department acknowledged declining participation in its officially sanctioned group programs.[32] Autonomous weight-loss groups now overshadowed those managed under medical authority.

Probably the first program to take root outside the expert domain was called TOPS, which stands for "Take Off Pounds Sensibly." Begun in early 1948 by housewife and mother Esther Manz and a handful of like-minded Milwaukee area women, TOPS had been meeting regularly for a year before Rutstein proposed (perhaps independently) a group weight-loss approach in the Newton project. Inspired by her experience in a prenatal class run by her family doctor, as well as what she had heard about AA and the psychiatric understanding of obesity, Manz helped shape an approach that featured "competitive play" and elements borrowed from group psychotherapy.[33]

According to Parr, the TOPS understanding was that fat people ate as a coping mechanism when confronted by stressful and challenging situations and by negative emotions. Supposedly to strengthen the participant's ego so as to manage emotions and meet challenges differently, TOPS cultivated a playful attitude—from humorous chapter names (e.g., Alter Egos, Trim-a-Donnas, Classy Chassis) to the games incorporated into typical sessions, such as "calories baseball" (where members returned, or batted back, the calorie count of foods "pitched" to them). Such activities varied, but every chapter included a game-like "weigh-in" ritual at

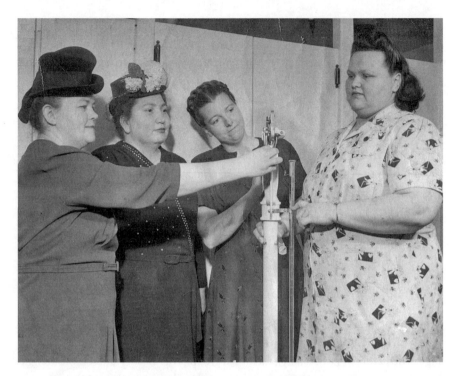

The weighing-in ritual with which each meeting of TOPS began, 1948. © TOPS Club Inc.

the opening of each meeting in which every participant's progress was assessed and announced. Spinning-top badges were given to those who had lost weight, turtle badges to those who had neither lost nor gained, and pig badges to those who had gained weight. The "pigs" would contribute money (five cents typically) to the piggy bank and be required to perform a debasing ritual, such as wearing a pig bib, sitting in a mock pigpen, oinking when pointed at, or singing a "pig song" (e.g., "We are plump little pigs who ate too much fat, fat, fat / We are stout little pigs who ate too much food, food, food," to the tune of "The Whiffenpoof Song"). There followed a mock trial in a "court of weight and measures" where those who had gained would confess their failings in detail, and constructive input might be offered by others (which might be practical advice, emotional support, or behavioral suggestions). Obviously, stigma and the associated shame and guilt from a failure of self-control were harnessed as motivators. A few elements of TOPS practice were borrowed from AA, such as reliance on a pairing system of "reducing pals," the use of somber pledges, and the framing of weight loss as a lifetime commitment. Unlike some other groups, however, there was no counterpart in TOPS to the Twelve Steps and no overt spirituality. Chapters of the organization spread rapidly through the midwestern United States in the early 1950s, and by 1965 the organization had reached every state, with a national membership of several hundred thousand.[34]

A contrasting approach that was at least as popular among nonmedical weight-loss groups relied not on games or other social interactions, but fundamentally on introspection and spiritual renewal. Rutstein had alluded to Alcoholics Anonymous when he first proposed group weight loss in Newton, and in doing so he showed awareness of current psychiatric thinking that went beyond just the oral fixation theory of obesity attributed to Hilde Bruch. Offering a mutual aid model with evangelical roots, AA had attracted great interest among psychiatrists in the 1940s for its success in managing a previously intractable addiction, despite its frankly spiritual and seemingly irrational elements. Bill W., AA's cofounder, was invited as a keynote speaker to the 1949 American Psychiatric Association meeting; mental hospitals imitated AA in their group therapy for alcoholics and released patients into community AA programs; and AA was studied by some psychotherapists as a source of techniques and insights into alcoholism.[35] Alcoholics Anonymous and its Twelve Steps also became widely known to the American public after the *Saturday Evening Post* ran a piece on the program in 1941, which fueled the fellowship's growth. By about 1950, AA had spread throughout the nation and begun to diversify to other addictive conditions, spawning Narcotics Anonymous and Alateen (for the children of alcoholics).[36]

Alcoholics Anonymous used medical-sounding language to frame alcoholism as a disease—thus reducing moral judgment and stigma around the condition—but did so in a way that varied greatly from the dominant psychiatric understanding of addiction as an oral fixation. Instead, in a construal that outran scientific plausibility, AA claimed that alcoholics differed from healthy individuals in having an idiosyncratic physical reaction to alcohol, sometimes described as an allergy, such that alcohol exerted a uniquely destructive and irresistible effect on them. For this reason, the first of AA's Twelve Steps was to admit that one is powerless over alcohol, so that complete abstention from drinking is the only way forward. This raised obvious problems for adapting AA's approach to the problem of overeating, since it is not possible to abstain from food entirely. The subsequent—frankly spiritual—steps were more easily adapted to overeating and other "defects" framed as addictions. Participants in Twelve Step programs sought help and forgiveness from a Higher Power, made amends to those they have harmed, and conducted a "searching and fearless moral inventory" and a continuing "personal inventory" of their own character. In this respect, the goal of Twelve Step programs corresponds at least partly to the insights sought in psychoanalysis.[37]

Weight-loss groups based on the AA model incorporated other now-familiar aspects of the approach. Meetings centered on sharing embarrassing experiences or shameful confessions, and participants partnered with "sponsors" whom they could call in times of trouble. But a closer adaptation of the AA approach to weight loss took some time. An important early effort was Fatties Anonymous (FA), founded around 1950 by Ruth Douglas, an unmarried, college-educated New Yorker—thus different from the type of participant associated with groups like TOPS (described by contemporary observers as typically married and lower-middle or working class). Just as AA members must admit they are powerless over drink, Douglas insisted, "Fatties Anonymous members had to admit, first, that they are unable to resist food." Douglas issued the "Ten Commandments" for FA in place of the Twelve Steps, the first commandment being a solemn oath that "I will eat to live, not live to eat." Thus the quest for personal self-realization and fulfillment replaced or merged with traditional religious piety, as in the pastoral psychology that flourished in the United States of the 1950s.[38]

The remaining commandments required conscientious and unsparingly honest self-examination, combined with techniques designed to break engrained patterns of thought and behavior and replace them with what now would be called self-esteem:

2. I will eat sensibly, carefully.
3. While dieting I will submit to medical care.
4. I will get weighed every day.
5. I will keep a chart, recording what I have eaten and at what time and how many calories consumed.
6. I will read one new book every month, one that will give me an inspiring viewpoint on life.
7. I will make a conscious effort to understand myself, weighing my finding[s] honestly, accentuating my good points and minimizing or overcoming my faults.
8. I will observe one DSD [do something different] day each week. Go some place never before visited, listen to a new program, wear my hair differently, try a new recipe. I will exert myself to do one new thing, no matter how trivial, tho [*sic*] it only means coming home a different way.
9. I will make at least one new friend or acquaintance each month.

10. To cultivate my sense of awareness, I will study other people, how they affect me and why, how I affect them; study what they've got and what I've got but [not?] where I miss.

At FA meetings, much as in AA, individual confessions took center stage. At one meeting, for example, a woman explained how her husband had left her for another woman because of the "shiftless, untidy eating frump he had to come home to." Another described cracking under the strain of remaining "merry . . . around the house" to keep her husband's interest despite her "tent-size" clothing. According to Douglas, one of the key benefits for participants was hearing the "same old alibis and defenses" coming from the mouths of others. This experience and other "know thyself revelations" helped the participant understand how "silly" and baseless her own excuses were. The twin goals of the program were to help participants achieve awareness and perhaps resolution of the "inner conflicts" driving overeating, while simultaneously receiving help with designing and sticking with a diet. Despite considerable press exposure and strong initial interest, however, FA seems not to have survived the mid-1950s, possibly due to unstable leadership.[39]

The group Overeaters Anonymous (OA) picked up where FA left off. Rozanne S., a middle-aged mother and housewife, started OA in the Los Angeles area around the beginning of 1960 because she could not find a local group to help her fight her late-night binge eating. Rozanne brought a familiarity with Twelve Step programs to the initiative, having previously attended open Gamblers Anonymous meetings. Accordingly, OA adheres more tightly to the AA formula than did FA, offering a Twelve Step program that explicitly invokes a Higher Power: "God as we understand him." Unlike either TOPS or FA, OA observes strict anonymity. Still more introspective than FA, OA does not dwell on the details of reducing diets, weigh its members, or encourage competition. The group achieved fairly wide reach by the late 1960s, with thousands of members nationally. Like TOPS, OA continues to offer programming today on a nonprofit basis.[40]

Much more than TOPS, the groups modeled on AA prioritize internal, psychological change; the goal is reflective insight and, through acceptance, psychological transformation—even "rebirth." Others, however, built on the idea that people should work on changing their behavior rather than changing themselves. This latter approach lends itself particularly well to commercialization. The most famous of these behaviorally oriented programs is Weight Watchers, founded in 1961 by Jean Nidetch, a charismatic, overweight New York housewife who was having trouble adhering to a medically endorsed diet. Weight Watchers started out as a group-therapy-inspired club involving half a dozen of Nidetch's "fat friends," with an emphasis on food choice and how to stick with a diet. In 1963, seeing herself and others lose weight through her brand of mutual support, Nidetch incorporated to promote and profit from her successful formula.[41]

Nidetch's business success is based on local chapters' fidelity to the formula, and all meeting leaders are successful former participants. Meetings resemble health education classes at least as much as group psychotherapy. Each begins with a private weigh-in for every participant, which is followed by a lecture and then an open experience-sharing discussion moderated by the leader. Weight Watchers particularly focuses on dieting techniques and tips (for example, washing a cookie like a fruit whenever struck with the urge to eat one) and provides participants with very specific menus requiring that ingredients be weighed. By early 1967 Weight Watchers was offering 297 classes per week in the New York City area alone. The organization claimed "25 franchise operations in 16 states" as well as in London and Tel Aviv and boasted many celebrity enthusiasts; by 1968, it had a million members. When the company floated shares on the stock market that year, Nidetch became a millionaire. A decade later, the company was purchased by the food multinational Heinz.[42] Obviously, weight-loss groups whose primary mode was introspection offered less opportunity for profit. In any case, whether the meetings were intro- spective or behaviorally oriented, millions of Americans participated in nonmed- ical, mutually assisted weight-loss groups during the 1950s and 1960s.

An Enormously Successful Failure

Public health originally embraced group weight-loss programs as an individu- alistic, cheap, politically innocuous alternative to mass heart disease screening pro- grams. The intervention soon proved so successful, however, that the groups orga- nized by health departments could not compete with the autonomous clubs that proliferated in YWCAs and church basements across the country. That group weight loss proved so popular among American women in the 1950s owes much to factors having little to do with physical health. Given the regular references to "moral support" and fellowship as an experience of group participation, it would not be very speculative to suggest that one benefit was social, helping relieve any loneliness or sense of isolation that participants may have felt from being fat or simply from being housewives in suburbia. To the extent that group weight-loss programs met psychosocial needs and perhaps mitigated obesity-related health harms like diabetes among participating women, it may be regarded as a modest success (keeping in mind that diabetes was an order of magnitude less important as a cause of death than heart disease, even among women).[43]

As a public health intervention in the fight against heart disease, however, group weight-loss programs must be considered a failure. The approach was conceived by public health leaders like Rutstein as a way of fighting heart disease, but since heart disease mortality was highest (and increasing) among men, men would have had to participate in great numbers. However, the evidence strongly suggests that participants were overwhelmingly white, middle-class women. According to Harvard nutritionist Jean Mayer in the mid-1960s, this was the type of American who least needed to lose weight, because "social pressure" kept it down—pressure that was "very class sensitive with obesity much more prevalent among lower than among upper classes." He judged obesity to be much more of a problem for white men (apparently of all classes) and "colored" women, because social pressure to be slim was lacking among both groups. As for "colored" men, Mayer believed that obesity was not a big problem because "they do most of the physical work that needs to be done around the place." (Based on the National Health Examination Survey of 1959–1962, discussed in chapter 6, Mayer's optimism about the obesity-related health condition of white women fits with their better blood pressure levels at all ages and slightly better glucose tolerance under fifty compared with black women, but his optimism about black men was misplaced. They fared worse than white men both in blood pressure at all ages and in glucose tolerance over sixty.)[44] Whatever benefits that white women derived, the voluntarism of this public health intervention meant that it did not affect those who needed it most.

Group weight-loss programs, in other words, represent a classic hands-off or, perhaps better, "hidden hand" approach in which the government offers little central planning or direction, instead acting by stimulating private initiative.[45] This is not to say that President Dwight Eisenhower was actively opposed to public health measures during his 1950s reign—far from it. When, for example, House Republicans attempted to gut the Food and Drug Administration by slashing its staff and budget, Eisenhower and his secretary of health, education, and welfare, Oveta Culp Hobby, saved the agency by organizing a friendly citizens review committee featuring pharmaceutical executives and other business heavyweights who perceived the need for stable regulation.[46] Eisenhower even left Truman's surgeon general, Leonard Scheele, in office, favoring continuity and professionalism over partisan loyalties. The former general simply had other priorities—the most important being prosecution of the Cold War, a task that Eisenhower took deadly seriously.

Unfortunately, as public health leaders lamented in the mid-1950s, with 65 percent of federal revenue allocated to military spending, 10 percent to servicing the national debt, and 7 percent to veterans' benefits, the Department of Health, Education, and Welfare was lucky if it came away with 1 percent. And only a sliver of that went to public health.[47] There was, however, one occasion when the Eisenhower administration took a special interest in an issue central to the fight against obesity.

Fighting Shape

Eisenhower—known as "Ike" to friends and detractors alike—believed in exercise. A keen football player in his youth, he conspicuously golfed during his presidency. His experience as a military leader had taught him sports' importance both for physical fighting capability and for morale. It was with alarm, then, that he received the news from Republican senator James Duff in 1955 that American children had fallen drastically behind their European counterparts in fitness.[48]

Duff's message concerned a 1954 study conducted by Hans Kraus and Ruth Prudden Hirschland (remembered now as Bonnie Prudden, a founder of modern rock climbing), two physical education researchers based in New York. Kraus and Prudden compared a large sample of American and European (Austrian, Italian, and Swiss) schoolchildren aged six to sixteen on various performance measures designed to test what they called "minimum muscular fitness." The study did not assess obesity levels in children; rather, it was designed to "determine whether or not the individual has sufficient strength and flexibility in the parts of the body upon which demands are made in normal daily living." The highly standardized test rated children's ability to make certain basic movements, such as touching the floor while standing with legs straight or rolling up from a lying to a seated position. The American and European children were all healthy and comparable in terms of age, economic bracket, and community backgrounds, but the differences were striking: only one in ten of the European children failed one or more of the fitness tests, compared with more than half of the Americans. American children attending rural and private schools performed somewhat better, leading the authors to conclude that exercise was protective and that mechanization, especially in transportation, was largely to blame for the shocking finding of national unfitness.[49]

Eisenhower was reportedly "appalled" by this discovery, noting its connection to the worrying fact that more than half of the 4 million men drafted for the armed forces since 1948 had failed their preinduction medical examinations. Media reports echoed his alarm, reinforcing the idea that something was deeply wrong with America's children. National magazines explained that a "rich diet," modern conveniences, and passive television entertainment—"life by gadget"—were making youth "soft," "fat and flabby." Given the public health community's concerns about obesity, one might expect federal authorities to have evaluated reports of declining fitness among children as yet another sign that Americans were getting too fat. But childhood obesity does not seem to have been explicitly discussed by either government or media sources. For Eisenhower, it was all about the Cold War. Apart from the issue of maintaining a military force physically capable of fighting, there were two distinct but related problems. First, the lack of physical fitness among youth, presumed to stem from television and modern conveniences, signaled that Americans might be *morally* unprepared for the lengthy global struggle with communism. The easy luxuries of postwar life had made Americans lazy and comfortable. As Shane McCarthy, the initial head of Eisenhower's response to the crisis, put it, "The nation that has been sleeping soundly on soft cushions may wake up dead."[50] Thus, the opposite of "fit" for the Eisenhower administration was not "fat" but "soft." Many media outlets echoed the softness theme. *Newsweek*, for instance, titled an early feature on the problem of childhood fitness "Are We Becoming Soft?" As many historians of the Cold War have noted, midcentury Americans displayed a phobia of effeminate "softness" (as opposed to striving, masculine "hardness") as a sign of vulnerability to communist infiltration.[51]

The second indirect threat of the lack of fitness of American youth relates to the ongoing struggle for cultural prestige between the United States and the Soviet Union and therefore for legitimacy in world leadership as perceived by other nations. The cultural Cold War, as historians describe this struggle for prestige, was fought on many fronts, including the arts, literature, science, and sports.[52] That athletic achievement was a front in the Cold War became evident in early 1956 when the Soviet Union under Nikita Khrushchev took the most medals at the winter Olympics in Cortina, Italy. Eisenhower's archived office files contain many newspaper and magazine clippings on the Olympics, testifying to his surprise and dismay at how America's athletes had been outshone. A February 1956 feature in *U.S. News and World Report* expressed grave concern about the coming summer Olympics in Melbourne, Australia. The piece put the problem succinctly: "Soviet sport champions are turning out to be effective propagandists for Communism. . . . Their victories are boosting Soviet prestige around the world." After noting the system of compulsory sports education in Soviet schools, the article concluded by mildly suggesting that some government funding ought to be provided for the US

Olympic teams—lest the Olympics continue to supply the world with evidence of "American 'decadence.'"[53]

By the time of the summer Olympics, the Eisenhower administration had sprung into action. On July 11, 1955, soon after he first heard reports of the children's fitness study, Eisenhower had convened a lunchtime conference at the White House. The researchers presented their alarming finding to more than thirty "sports leaders," including former boxing champion Gene Tunney, baseball star Willie Mays, and college basketball sensation Bill Russell. Notable officials present included the presidents of the US Olympic Committee and the Amateur Athletic Union. The administration soon laid plans for the Conference on the Fitness of American Youth, to be held that September under the chairmanship of Vice President Richard Nixon. Attendees would meet to discuss the nation's physical fitness situation and seek ways to improve it. Ironically, the conference had to be rescheduled after the president suffered a heart attack a few days beforehand.

Eisenhower recuperated under the care of Paul Dudley White, to the delight and benefit of American cardiologists. Meanwhile, the planners of the conference—which finally took place in June 1956—issued a series of recommendations calling for cooperation among all levels of education and amateur sports organizations, especially at the community level. The conference planners called on "television, radio, and other media to tell the story of fitness" and asked federal, state, and local governments to fund "demonstration projects to dramatize the steps to and the fitness of youth." To help implement these measures, Eisenhower established the President's Council on Youth Fitness (PCYF), headed by Shane McCarthy and made up of representatives from thirty-five federal agencies. The separate Citizens Advisory Committee on the Fitness of American Youth included prominent businessmen and the type of "sports leader" included at the luncheon. But in keeping with Eisenhower's approach to both public health and governing in general, there would be no "overriding Federal program"; the project was diverse, local, voluntary, and open-ended. And not much federal money was spent on it.[54]

The great bulk of the activities associated with the PCYF focused on promoting physical fitness without any explicit connection to diet, obesity, or even health—perhaps unsurprising in this context, given that "fitness" had been constructed chiefly as a military and moral problem. One typical set of PCYF recommendations urged schools to keep their playgrounds open after hours and during summer vacations and suggested that cities close certain streets regularly to allow safe outdoor play in the absence of adequate playgrounds. The PCYF also promulgated calisthenics programs for primary schools lacking organized sports and proper facilities (as most public schools did). The National Youth Fitness Week program stimulated and showcased local initiatives.[55]

A handful of PCYF activities and recommendations did, however, touch directly on the domain of public health. For example, Prudden, now a member of the youth fitness advisory committee, urged a women's club audience to exercise to reduce their own flab. But, she reminded them, they also had a responsibility to make their children fit to fight and to "get your husbands moving [or] they will die"—largely from heart disease, as she noted elsewhere.[56] But like the group weight-loss programs, children's fitness programs during the Eisenhower years cannot be viewed as a substantial contribution to public health, except perhaps indirectly in that some children who were encouraged to bicycle, play Little League, and so forth may have maintained those physical activity habits into adulthood.

When John F. Kennedy assumed the presidency in 1961, he rebranded the youth fitness group as the President's Council on Physical Fitness in hopes of bringing adults under its purview. Kennedy's council took a more regimented and directive approach to fitness than had Eisenhower's by, for example, issuing standardized gymnastics drills for schools through the Department of Education. The administration spent considerable money publicizing and promoting its "Official U.S. Physical Fitness Program." But despite its deliberate inclusion of American adults, who were consistently imagined as flabby and listless, the council in the 1960s did not make weight control a special priority any more than it had under Eisenhower.[57]

Why were federal authorities in the late 1950s and 1960s so uninterested in addressing the obesity epidemic perceived by Dublin and other public health leaders around 1950? Certainly not because of any evidence that Americans were in general losing weight. Indeed, there was good evidence that Americans were growing ever heavier. But cardiologists and other medical researchers were increasingly unsure that obesity contributed directly to heart disease. And if obesity did not cause heart disease, why fight it, especially when other avenues of intervention were opening, such as drugs for hypertension and cholesterol-lowering diets? Such questions would trouble public health authorities for the next two decades.

CHAPTER 5

The New Epidemiology and Its Impact

In 1962 the CBS television network aired a high-profile program entitled *The Fat American*, hosted by ace newsman Harry Reasoner and featuring a firmament of scientific stars. Its theme: the United States was killing itself with its own success. "One out of three adult Americans are overweight" thanks, intoned Reasoner, to "progress that has brought abundance; progress that has brought a sharp decline in drudgery." Snippets from interviews with the scientists underscored the sense of danger and decadence. Paul Dudley White said, "One hundred percent of Americans, practically, eat too much," stuffing themselves like Roman aristocrats. Thomas Dawber, the Framingham study's chief investigator, revealed that men who gained 20 percent over their weight at age twenty-five suffered double the rate of coronary disease as men who did not. And Jean Mayer warned of skyrocketing childhood obesity. Asked Reasoner in conclusion, was not "the way we eat" increasingly a "matter of life and death"?[1]

About fifteen years later Ancel Keys, the famed physiologist and expert on heart disease—and a promoter of the "Mediterranean diet"—once again conjured the fat American before a popular audience. Whenever he and his wife return from Italy to the United States, he began, "we are struck by the many extremely fat people we see." "All these near-monsters walking around" explain why "there is such a flourishing reducing industry." But he ended with a twist. After a lengthy attack on the insurance industry's studies, which he held responsible for the idea that overweight shortened people's lifespan, he gave news that the average American would welcome: the latest "truly scientific studies," such as his own, showed that for middle-aged men, "20 pounds in the middle of the weight distribution has little or no health significance." Essentially, being a bit overweight was not unhealthy; weight was only a matter of aesthetic concern except in extreme cases; and the weight-loss industry was just a psychologically brutal scam.[2] While nobody else among the community of heart disease experts was as outspokenly skeptical about obesity as Keys, by the

1970s his permissive attitude had become mainstream. Most agreed that *how much* we eat did not matter as much as *what* we eat.

This shift in the climate of opinion had to do with early evidence emerging from the first generation of prospective community studies, such as Framingham, which quantified the importance of obesity and other factors as predictors of heart disease. Hypertension retained its preeminence as a risk factor, but obesity lost its leading place to serum cholesterol, and for a time overweight became just a secondary risk factor in the minds of many epidemiologists. The shift also had to do with funding sources, laboratory science, and the introduction around 1960 of prescription drugs that made lowering blood pressure a more convenient way for doctors to manage heart disease risk than reducing body weight. Around the same time, special diets did the same for serum cholesterol, and cholesterol drugs followed. Thus, as a medical matter, while obesity remained a target in the war against heart disease, it grew increasingly less preferred; by the end of the 1960s, calls to control Americans' weight had lost their urgency. As I show in chapter 6, American society changed too, such that the "monstrous" bodies of the obese no longer triggered the same sense of threat.

New Theories from New Data

Coronary heart disease accounted for a third of US deaths in the 1950s, the situation seemed worst among white males, and the death toll was rising, at least among them.[3] This understanding of the problem carried through the next decade. The preferred responses to the heart disease epidemic drew on an evolving body of science that attempted to discover the causes of CHD. Framingham was only the most famous of a clutch of prospective studies seeking to realize White's postwar dream of a multiyear heart disease study that would survey the health of "entire communities" or at least population samples. Especially in the 1960s, this first generation of prospective CHD studies generated new methods for inferring causes from statistical associations: the researchers at Framingham, for example, developed new methods for analyzing the associations between multiple variables, which revolutionized epidemiology.[4] Collectively, these well-regarded studies cast doubt on obesity as a leading driver of heart disease in the United States.

Before discussing the specific findings, it is worth pausing for a moment to consider how these studies differed from the life insurance studies that had previously established obesity as a scourge of public health. Proponents of the major prospective studies pointed out that they represented truer samples of the general population than those found in insurance records. While a valid criticism, it is also the case that the insurance industry studies were based on millions of people, samples two or three orders of magnitude larger than the new longitudinal surveys. Furthermore, the fact that insured people were unusually free of known health problems only made them better subjects for investigating the predictive value of specific conditions, such as high blood pressure and weight, in contributing to later heart disease. The best lab mice are, after all, carefully bred to be more uniform than wild animals. It is thus in some ways surprising that most epidemiologists and cardiologists so wholeheartedly embraced the newer surveys over the previous insurance study data, which showed obesity to be one of, if not the chief, driver of heart disease mortality.

The Framingham researchers had chosen a whole (mostly white) town and evaluated most of the population within a certain age bracket, but not all of the other prospective heart disease studies born at the same time followed suit. Some more closely resembled the insurance company studies—albeit on a smaller scale—in that they followed a sample cohort of healthy and supposedly typical people, especially the white middle-class men about whom politicians showed the greatest concern, over time. Some of these studies, moreover, were specifically designed to highlight individual risk factors thought to contribute to coronary heart disease. Besides the obvious and well-established risk factors of obesity and high blood pressure, laboratory studies had implicated high-fat diets and serum cholesterol. Several other plausible causes had been advanced sufficiently to merit examination in the cohort studies, including an anxiety-prone personality, cigarette smoking, and lack of physical exercise. Thus, most of the first-wave prospective studies of the causes of CHD addressed some combination of variables that included blood pressure, obesity, serum cholesterol, anxiety, smoking, and physical activity.

Ancel Keys was associated with many of the important studies that suggested a more prominent role for dietary fats than obesity in CHD. Known for his forceful opinions and self-assurance, the University of Minnesota professor began a small prospective study on volunteer white "businessmen" in 1947. Keys's colleague Henry Blackburn later recalled this study as "vastly underpowered" and indicative of the researchers' naïveté, in that statistical analyses require a much larger sample than 300 individuals to demonstrate anything but the most dramatic differences in outcome frequency.[5] Over the ensuing decades, Keys built his statistical sophistication while maintaining his unwavering conviction that body weight had little to do with heart disease.

Based on the insight that because muscle weighs more than fat, physically fit

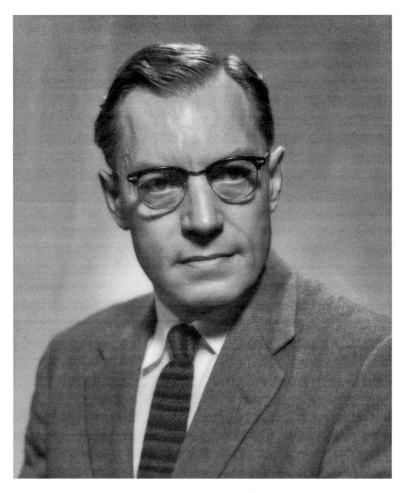

University of Minnesota physiology professor Ancel Keys, 1950s. Courtesy of University of Minnesota Archives, University of Minnesota, Twin Cities.

men, like professional football players, were heavier than average yet still healthier, Keys evidently designed the 1947 study to show that exercise was at least as important as weight. From the group of about 1,000 Minneapolis men who initially responded to his advertisements, Keys and his co-investigators chose 50 who were markedly underweight, 50 who were markedly overweight, 50 who were purportedly very physically active, and 150 others at random. Each participant received a physical examination that included measurements of blood pressure, serum cholesterol, body fat percentage, and of course weight and height; these examinations were repeated regularly. The findings from this study were meager. After fifteen years, Keys determined that the handful of "businessmen" who had died of CHD had higher levels of cholesterol than those who remained alive. He also found that "men who develop coronary heart disease in spite of having relatively low serum choles-terol values are men who tend to be at the upper extremes of blood pressure or relative body weight, or both."[6]

His theories did not wait for these data, however. For reasons perhaps related to his war work on starvation (but still not entirely clear), Keys had already become convinced that particular patterns of food consumption could profoundly influ-ence people's metabolism, and he saw disordered fat metabolism as the prime cause of heart disease.[7] With Keys's commitment to explaining heart disease through qualitatively abnormal metabolism came a hostility to alternative explanations, especially obesity. For example, in one 1953 medical talk he lampooned what he saw as the moralistic attitudes toward fat people implicit in current public health campaigns like Metropolitan's, likening them to the "indignation formerly aroused by the man who insisted on putting his privy next to the well" and criticizing the "full steam ahead . . . campaign against overweight" among public health workers who had leaped to the conclusion that the greater obesity rate of the United States compared to other countries explains its greater age-specific mortality rate from heart disease. He liked to point out flaws in the insurance data, especially that in-surance examinations measured height and weight with shoes and indoor clothing on. It does not seem to have occurred to Keys that such errors in measuring fatness by clothed weight and height would only have blurred the data and therefore did not create but only obscured the consistently strong correlations between relative weight and heart disease mortality found in large insurance studies; that is, his crit-icism about the data actually supported the overweight–heart disease association. And that was not his only spurious argument.[8]

Like some other researchers who questioned the link between obesity and heart disease, including Fred Stare, Keys's intellectual commitments may have been re-lated to his funders. Several medical writers, most notably Cristin Kearns and Gary Taubes, have established that like Stare, Keys received significant funding from the sugar industry beginning in the mid-1940s. He also was funded by the tobacco in-dustry in the early 1950s. Sugar consumption, of course, was thought to be a major factor in weight gain. Through the Sugar Research Foundation, the industry hoped to deflect attention onto dietary fats as the heart disease culprit and to capture whatever share of the American diet that fatty foods (meat, dairy products) lost for "the carbohydrate industries." The tobacco industry presumably backed Keys's efforts to demonstrate a link between dietary fat and heart disease as part of its larger strategy of using science to deflect attention away from cigarette smoking as a cause of cancer and heart disease. The tobacco industry does not seem to have funded Keys for long, based on an expert biostatistician's assessment of his work as "sketchy" and lacking in analytical rigor, but his sugar funding lasted at least until 1970.[9] In any case, it is impossible to say whether Keys's convictions about the causes of heart disease attracted his industry funding or if the funding informed his convictions.

In the 1950s Keys's contention that diet composition (focusing on fat, especially particular fats) rather than quantity (calories) was the prime cause of America's heart disease problem rested not on his own prospective epidemiological research, but mainly on a different type of study. These studies compared the average serum cholesterol levels, dietary fat intake (inferred from typical consumption patterns and gross economic data), and heart disease rates (from death certificate data) in different countries or groups. For example, in one influential 1953 article summarizing his argument, Keys showed that CHD death rates for men correlated closely with average serum cholesterol levels and total dietary fat intake across samples from Minnesota, Naples, London, and both rich and poor residents of Madrid (who had high and low heart mortality, respectively). Obesity levels, whether measured by weight and height tables or by body fat percentages, did not correlate so well with death rates; indeed, Naples had a comparable obesity prevalence to Minneapolis but much lower heart disease mortality. In a similar study, this one undermining the role of heredity in favor of diet, Keys found that Japanese men living in Japan, where coronary disease rates and dietary fat intake were both low, had low serum cholesterol, while Japanese American men in Hawaii and Los Angeles showed much higher serum cholesterol and CHD mortality.[10]

Again, these studies did not assess the diets of the actual individuals whose blood was tested. This is a major reason that Keys's work relating both fat consumption and serum cholesterol levels to coronary heart disease on the national and group level was not universally respected. (Indeed, it was this type of study that the tobacco consultant, Harvard statistician Edwin Wilson, found shoddy.) Apart from the obvious limitations involving death certificate completion practices, the questionable quality of diet information, and countless other confounding variables, it was possible to use the same international data to demonstrate a stronger correlation of national heart disease mortality with sugar intake and gross caloric intake than with fat intake. Perhaps unsurprisingly, the researcher who showed this—British physiologist John Yudkin, himself funded heavily by the dairy industry—became Keys's archnemesis from the mid-1950s through the 1960s.[11]

Other researchers with different commitments also launched prospective epidemiological studies around the same time as Keys's businessmen project. In 1949 public health researchers with the state and city departments of health in Los Angeles launched a longitudinal study that involved about 2,200 middle-aged male civil servants. All these subjects were given a general physical and cardiological examination, which was repeated every twelve to eighteen months. Early findings from Los Angeles available during the 1950s included strong evidence that employees with relatively sedentary jobs tended to die of CHD more often, as did highly overweight men and those with high blood pressure. This evidence of course tended to reinforce the already widespread belief that obesity, high blood pressure, and possibly lack of exercise (which might act by promoting overweight) were leading causes of heart disease.[12]

In 1953, New York state initiated a similar prospective study of heart disease among its civil servants. About 1,800 middle-aged Albany men underwent a physical and cardiological examination and then were regularly reexamined at roughly twelve-month intervals. By the time of the examination in late 1956, enough men had developed new ischemic heart disease (that is, CHD, defined slightly differently) to reveal a few significant predictors. Men with the highest serum cholesterol levels were nearly six times more prone to the disease than those with the lowest levels, and men who were the most overweight—40 percent or more over the actuarial ideal weight—were three times as prone as those who were less overweight. There was no correlation with job classification, perhaps because all were fairly sedentary; nor, surprisingly, was there any correlation with high blood pressure. When the results of the fourth examination became available in 1959, they reinforced the previous findings that both high cholesterol and marked overweight predisposed men to develop heart disease, and high blood pressure had also emerged as a significant risk factor. The Albany study additionally found that heavy smokers were twice as likely to develop heart disease than nonsmokers were, but the numbers were not yet sufficient to reach statistical significance. Similar studies across the country produced similar results.[13]

Thus, in the second half of the 1950s, several large prospective studies confirmed that high blood pressure and marked obesity predicted the development of coronary disease. Although the evidence was slightly weaker, these studies also demonstrated correlations between new CHD and high serum cholesterol, milder degrees of overweight, and smoking. All these studies played a role in establishing experts' consensus on the causes of CHD in the 1960s, but the one that counted most was Framingham.

The New Gold Standard: Framingham

The findings of the Framingham study shaped the ways that doctors and public health authorities have approached the problem of coronary heart disease from the late 1950s to the present day. As with the Albany and Los Angeles studies, the Framingham researchers published their first analysis of the factors that predisposed healthy adults to CHD in 1957. Of the nearly 900 men between forty-five and sixty-two years old initially enrolled in the study, 52 had developed the disease or had died suddenly of it after four years, providing a large enough sample to draw several statistically significant conclusions. The most robust findings underlined the role of high blood pressure in heart attacks: men with very high blood pressure were three to four times more likely to develop CHD than those with normal blood pressure, and those with "borderline" elevated blood pressure were more than twice as likely. High levels of serum cholesterol increased risk almost as strongly: men with the highest cholesterol on the initial examination were three times more likely to develop CHD than those with the lowest cholesterol. The researchers assumed that those with the highest levels of education would have the most sedentary lifestyles, but education level made no difference in the likelihood that a given participant developed heart disease. Smoking did not prove to be a statistically significant predictor in this first four-year period either, although the heaviest smokers did have the highest rates of CHD.[14]

At first glance, the initial findings seemed to support the link between obesity and coronary heart disease. Men in the top 10 percent of weight for their height (judged by reference to the community median, an index called the Framingham relative weight) were 2.5 times more likely to develop CHD than those of median weight. Those with lesser degrees of overweight had intermediate degrees of risk. As the 1957 report put it, "The present experience confirms the widespread belief that obesity is associated with the development of [CHD]."[15]

Upon closer analysis, however, the findings regarding obesity were more ambiguous. The investigators noted that many obese people also had elevated levels of cholesterol and blood pressure, confounding conclusions about the independent predictive power of each factor. Were the heaviest people developing more heart disease because they were fat or because they also had high blood pressure? In the

Table 12—Incidence of ASHD in Four-Year Follow-Up, Males 45–62 Classified According to Level of Blood Pressure, Relative Weight or Cholesterol Level (Effect of Other Variables Partly Controlled)

Blood Pressure	Attributes * Relative Weight	Total Cholesterol	Population at Risk	New Disease	Rate/1,000
All persons †			877	51	58
Classified on blood pressure (men with high relative weight or high cholesterol omitted):					
High	Med. or low	Med. or low	91	9	100
Borderline	Med. or low	Med. or low	242	9	37
Normotension	Med. or low	Med. or low	240	4	17
Classified on relative weight (men with high blood pressure or high cholesterol omitted):					
Border. or normo.	High	Med. or low	87	5	57
Border. or normo.	Medium	Med. or low	198	5	25
Border. or normo.	Low	Med. or low	284	8	28
Classified on cholesterol (men with high blood pressure or high relative weight omitted):					
Border. or normo.	Med. or low	High	112	9	80
Border. or normo.	Med. or low	Medium	178	9	51
Border. or normo.	Med. or low	Low	304	4	13

* Classification of attributes:
  Blood pressure
    High—consistently 160 systolic or over or 100 diastolic or over
    Normotension—consistently below 140 systolic and 90 diastolic
    Borderline high blood pressure—all other
  Relative weight
    High—Framingham relative weight 113 or over
    Medium—Framingham relative weight 100–112
    Low—Framingham relative weight under 100
  Total cholesterol
    High—260 mg per cent or over
    Medium 225–259 mg per cent
    Low—under 225 mg per cent
  † Excludes 21 persons for (one developing new disease) whom measurements of one or more attributes were not available.

An early analysis of prospective data from the Framingham study supported the importance of obesity as a cause of heart disease. Reprinted from T. R. Dawber, Felix E. Moore, and George V. Mann, "II. Coronary Heart Disease in the Framingham Study," *American Journal of Public Health* 47 (1957): 4–24, table 12.

era before they had made their breakthroughs in multivariate statistical techniques, the Framingham investigators addressed this problem by looking in turn at men with elevated readings in only one of these three areas (that is, by stratification). Among men who were not obese and had low cholesterol, for example, those with very high blood pressure were six times more prone to heart disease than those with low blood pressure. The predictive power of high cholesterol alone was nearly as great when viewed in this way. But although obese men with low cholesterol and low blood pressure experienced CHD at twice the rate as similar men below median weight, the difference was not statistically significant.

Part of the problem here is that there were not many men high in weight but low in both cholesterol and blood pressure; larger numbers bring a given difference closer to statistical significance. More problematic for anyone expecting confirmation of the insurance studies, there was no difference at all between men at median weight and those below median (median weight in Framingham was well above actuarial ideal weight, as in the United States generally). As the four-year report concluded. "Apparently most of the association of risk of coronary disease with obesity is accounted for by the association of obesity with high blood pressure." Obesity skeptics like Keys pounced on the findings—even though the 1957 Framingham report made a point of supporting the general conclusions of life insurance studies on obesity and of criticizing a paper by Keys on hospital-based samples of heart attack patients, which showed no association with weight.[16] Since the Framingham study was intended to last twenty years, these 1957 findings were early, but they nevertheless would remain the gold standard for epidemiological evidence about obesity and other causes of CHD for another five years.

In 1959, the insurance industry essentially confirmed the new wisdom when it released a massive new multicompany study led by Metropolitan. The so-called Build and Blood Pressure study was based on an analysis of nearly 5 million insured people who were followed between 1935 and 1954. The study found that moderately elevated blood pressure alone was a much more dramatic contributor to excess mortality than moderate overweight alone; men had to be more than 25 percent above the average weight (not the ideal weight) to suffer a significant penalty. When combined with elevated blood pressure, however, milder overweight was much worse: "moderate overweight in combination with blood pressure of only the slightest upward departure from normal produces a mortality expectancy nearly twice the expected," wrote the lead author.[17]

Given that significantly overweight men almost always had at least slightly elevated blood pressure levels, the concrete implications for heart disease prevention were unchanged by the emerging doubt around obesity's status as a true cause. Fat men died early from heart disease, as Dawber had emphasized on CBS's *Fat American*. It would take until 1967, when twelve years' worth of data were analyzed, for the Framingham researchers to demonstrate a significant correlation between initial obesity, without high blood pressure or high cholesterol, and later sudden death from heart attack (and also angina, but not the composite, chief outcome measure of new CHD).[18] Not until 1988 did the Framingham investigators accumulate enough data to show a statistically significant elevated risk of new CHD for obesity even when not accompanied by high cholesterol and high blood pressure.[19]

In any case, even after all these studies had released their first sets of findings, obesity remained the most easily identified and, in theory, tractable cause of heart disease death. For that reason, clinical and public health attention remained focused on reducing obesity in the 1950s. In the 1960s, as blood pressure became more amenable to clinical intervention (more on this below), doctors gradually shifted their attention to hypertension. Indirect evidence, meanwhile, provided mounting support for the cholesterol metabolism theory of CHD, and diets that lowered serum cholesterol were available. Essentially, given the lack of epidemiological certainty around the three leading predictors of heart disease and the decreasing power of the resource-starved public health sector relative to the individual clinical services offered by America's 200,000 physician-businessmen, medical trends made obesity, blood pressure, and cholesterol fashionable in turn as targets for intervention.

Unhappy Doctors, Unhappy Patients

Mainstream doctors did not like fat patients. As the University of Pennsylvania psychologist Albert Stunkard, a pioneer in evaluating weight-loss approaches, put it in the CBS *Fat American* show, doctors thought that obesity was simple, a matter of more calories in than out, and that weight loss was equally simple: consume fewer calories. So they advised their patients to eat less and perhaps provided instructions for a reducing diet. And "yet the patient doesn't follow his advice, and then doctors tend to get very irritable and grouchy and sort of condemn the patients."[20] After all, if the patient who failed to lose weight was not at fault, then the doctor was. Many considered the woman who wanted to lose weight to be weak-willed or lazy and the man who needed to lose weight stubborn. In the 1950s the easiest way for the doctor to avoid such failure and to prevent heart disease or other obesity-related illness was to prescribe a pill that helped patients follow his excellent medical advice.

Throughout the 1950s and 1960s, the prescription diet pill of choice remained amphetamine. The drug had been introduced in the mid-1930s by the American firm Smith, Kline and French (SKF), initially as an antidepressant (the first of that class). Because of its appetite-suppressing side effects, specialists in the gray medical art of reducing quickly took up amphetamine as a diet pill, despite the fact it was not approved for weight loss until the late 1940s, when SKF ran controlled trials and began marketing it specifically for that purpose. Even before its patent on amphetamine expired in 1950, SKF had many competitors for the lucrative weight-loss market, both patent-infringing smaller firms selling amphetamine and other firms (small and large) selling methamphetamine, which is pharmacologically almost identical but was not protected by any patents. Throughout the 1950s, many drug firms poured marketing dollars into efforts to convince doctors to prescribe amphetamines liberally for weight loss.[21]

As I discussed in chapter 2, amphetamine diet pill advertising reinforced and amplified the new psychiatric stigma around overweight, capitalizing on the drug's established reputation as a psychiatric medication. Similarly, a good deal of prominent advertising reinforced and exploited the public health campaign against obesity launched by Metropolitan with support from the AMA and the PHS in 1951. One full-page SKF ad that ran in general medicine journals during June 1951 depicted the grossly swollen "liver of an OVERWEIGHT patient" suffering from heart disease (left ventricular hypertrophy with pulmonary edema) and insisted that "weight reduction—of even a few pounds—is often the surest means of lengthening life." An ad from 1953 was entitled "One Disease That Doesn't Hurt." It warned that unlike victims of most deadly illnesses, "the man who is 5 to 14 per cent overweight" will seldom complain if he "puff[s] a little at the top of the stairs," but "if his increasing weight is unchecked, he will become grossly obese" and suffer heart disease. Obesity was represented to doctors as an underdiagnosed, progressive, and deadly illness demanding aggressive therapy "while your patient is still in the marginal overweight class."[22] Thus in the 1950s the pharmaceutical industry played a part in disseminating among doctors recent scientific thinking, much of it stigmatizing, about overweight's causes and chronic disease consequences.

Since companies do not survive long if they badly misread their customers in their marketing efforts, it is worth going further in probing physician attitudes toward fat patients and obesity in diet pill advertising aimed at them. One popular marketing theme stressed that amphetamines support patients' willpower by reducing appetite. "Help her say 'no' when she's tempted to say 'yes,'" a 1953 pitch for Abbott's Desoxyn brand of methamphetamine put it. The text accompanied an illustration of a portly lady refusing a cake offered by a serpent during a social bridge game with three thin women. The implied relationship between doctor and patient here was sympathetic, in that the advertisement imagined a patient who wishes to cooperate with medical advice and needs her physician's help in doing so. Other marketing suggested a less supportive relationship. A 1955 ad for Massengill's

Medical journal advertising for prescription diet pills, almost all of which contained amphetamine, reinforced and exploited the early 1950s national public health campaign against obesity spearheaded by Metropolitan Life Insurance. Note how this ad encourages physicians to consider obesity a disease in itself, as well as seeing it as a cause of heart disease. Source: *Journal of the American Medical Association* 151, no. 1 (1953): 41.

Obedrin methamphetamine product, for example, made essentially the same major claim but pictured an adult cat in a posture of stern parental authority withholding a tempting fishbone, so that the kittens were forced to drink their milk.[23] Advertisements such as these positioned weight-loss drugs more as instruments for disciplining an immature patient than for helping a mature patient achieve her own goals.

Another Desoxyn ad, from 1960, illustrated a physician's disdain for patients who failed to comply with dietary advice by picturing a fat man of about sixty struggling to retrieve his wallet and shoes from the examining room floor. The doctor stands by, watching with arms folded and (seemingly) rolling eyes. An extreme example of this same attitude of annoyance and disrespect for fat, noncompliant patients can be found in a 1950 ad for Efroxine, a methamphetamine-based product from the small New Jersey firm Maltbie. In it, a plump, middle-aged, well-dressed woman, pictured as if across the desk from the doctor reading the ad, says, "Stick-to-it-iveness is fine—for everyone else . . . but take me. I just can't stick to my diet. I can't resist desserts." The text below asks: "If she thinks it's getting her down, what's it doing to physicians who have to listen to such explanations every day?" Whether sympathetic or condescending, all these ads underlined the medical community's assumption that their fat patients lacked strength of character. As medical professor Clifford Barborka put it at the 1951 AMA session launching Metropolitan's war on obesity, the fat patient typically did not have the "courage and perseverance" and to reduce food intake as medically advised—a lack driving many to seek a "quick and easy way" out in fads and quackery.[24] Barborka urged restraint in amphetamine prescribing, but to many doctors an approved medication to make patients compliant with medical instructions was better than the alternatives.

Prescription diet pill marketing invoked negative gender stereotypes. Advertisements depicting overweight women consistently expressed a general low regard toward them that transcended physicians' mere frustration with patients who resisted their authority. A common genre presented a woman vainly attempting to squeeze into an article of clothing too small for her; she is clearly unwilling to achieve her goals through virtuous abstention. A 1955 advertisement for Roerig's AmPlus amphetamine and vitamin combination, for example, features a two-panel cartoon. In the first panel—before treatment—a flabby young woman wearing a saggy one-piece swimsuit clasps a pair of skis unhappily. In the second panel—after treatment—the same woman appears thin, smiling, and cavorting on water

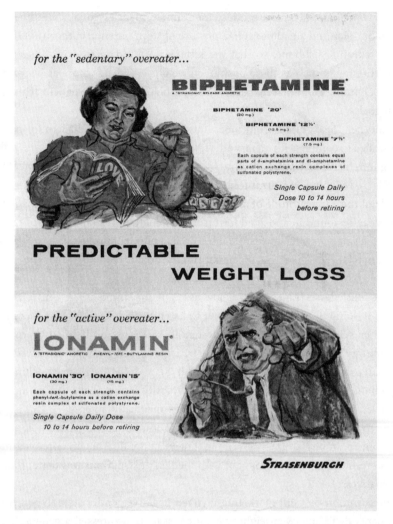

Medical journal advertising for prescription weight-loss medication shows a gendered difference in weight stigma, with women depicted as lazy, disengaged from active life, and/or psychiatrically disturbed. Source: *Journal of the American Medical Association* 174, no. 2 (1960): 35.

skis in a bikini. The title reads: "Prescription: AmPlus Now. Prognosis: Beachable by Summer." Another common stereotype was the couch-bound, middle-aged woman who finds fulfillment through eating rather than sexual satisfaction or worldly activity, as in the "sedentary overeater" indulging in chocolates while reading a magazine entitled *Love* in a 1960 ad for Strasenburgh's Biphetamine.[25]

The most common male stereotype in diet pill advertising and, by implication, in the physician's imagination was the hard-driving, fat businessman unwilling to acknowledge any need to care for his health. In a 1951 ad for Efroxine, for example, an elegantly dressed man of around sixty says, "I know you're right Doctor," "but I have too much else on my mind." "Yes it *is* quite a grind," the main text elaborated, "stocks and bonds, profits and losses, hurry and worry . . . no wonder your businessman patient finds it hard to live up to your diet instructions"—despite the fact that the doctor told him to lose weight "to ease the burden on his heart." Another example is Strasenburgh's depiction of the "'active' overeater" in a 1960 ad for its Ionamin amphetamine derivative: a fat, fiftyish man in a business suit talking and gesturing energetically while scarfing spaghetti.[26] Certainly this image is more sympathetic than that of the female chocolate-gobbling "'sedentary' overeater." Ads depicting men often mentioned heart disease and weight loss as a health measure rather than stressing vanity, the usual motive attributed to women (and not, for example, diabetes prevention).

For most doctors, obese people were difficult patients because they disrespected their physicians' dietary advice and wasted their time. There were certain doctors, however, who welcomed fat patients because they were cash cows. These "fat doctors," as they were often called by their mainstream fellows, or "bariatric practitioners," as they sometimes called themselves, did not enjoy much respect in the medical community. Other physicians frequently regarded them (with good reason) as quacks peddling remedies not far removed from the snake oil nostrums of the late nineteenth century. Typically these fat doctors directly dispensed the drugs they prescribed, cutting out the pharmacist and thus reaping huge profits.

Specialized drug firms produced pills, often in a wide range of colors, directly for this market. For example, Western Research Labs, a Denver-based supplier of "rainbow diet pills," sold doctors methamphetamine tablets as cheaply as $2 per thousand in the early 1960s, with the patients paying hundredfold markups. Western was already well established in 1948 when it first drew the attention of law enforcement after a patient died from taking the heart stimulant digitalis. At that time, the firm was also selling colorful pills containing digitalis, thyroid hormone, and the poison dinitrophenol (all of which had by then been declared dangerous and inappropriate for weight control) as well as addictive barbiturate sedatives. Some formulations offered many of these substances at once, combinations thought to help patients tolerate the stimulating effects of amphetamine, digitalis, and thyroid hormone. In addition to supplying weight-loss doctors with pills via a franchise system, Western provided clinics with additional materials, such as patient brochures. By 1958, when the firm again came to the FDA's attention, Western was thought to operate about 900 reducing practices and "salons" in the United States and Mexico.[27]

Western had competition from firms operating on similar business models, such as White Pharmacal, Mills, and Lanpar. All three of these companies manufactured the same types of colorful amphetamines and other more hazardous drugs for direct dispensing. Each also supplied weight loss doctors with educational materials and organized professional symposia that maintained an alternative universe of medical theory in which obesity was typically caused by glandular and heart dysfunction (rather than by psychologically driven overeating, as academic experts and medical textbooks all now agreed). A Lanpar brochure conveys the flavor of the practice and explains why the colors of the pills were important:

> Now, in building a weight reduction practice, there can be a quantity of good reception room gossip going on more or less behind your back, that will net you dollars from office patients. Now, many times in the office one girl on the desk will find a woman and they will talk weight reduction, she will get the history card out, she'll fill in the card, she'll have her already measured, her BP and pulse taken, and she'll have her sitting at your desk.
>
> Now you have to be situated with this reduction medicine. . . . You should have your selection of weight reduction medicine always complete so that you can cope with any situation that comes up, and you should have at least more than one color of every medication because here come two women in together. Do not give them the same color tablet. Don't let them go out and say "Well, all you've got to do is get these blue pills." Give one of them blue and one of them pink. After all it is individual medication for that patient. That's a little psychology and it is well worth it. Don't let the two women go out the door with the same color medicine.[28]

A fat doctor typically charged $10 to $40 per visit in the 1960s, and the visits were frequent (typically monthly) and short. A successful one might gross on average about $2,000 daily, seeing 100 patients "on a slow day." Lanpar alone counted about 1,150 physicians among its clients in the mid-1960s, when a congressional investigation threw a spotlight on the practice. According to that investigation, about 5,000 physicians nationally (many of them doctors of osteopathy) devoted the bulk of their practices to obesity, and 2,000 of these specialized strictly in weight loss. These practices earned $250 million annually just in patient fees, while their patients spent a conservatively estimated $120 million more on the medications they sold. Such patients consumed somewhere around 2 billion of the 8 billion pharmaceutical amphetamine tablets taken annually by Americans in the 1960s (the FDA's estimate of prescription amphetamine use changed little between the early and late 1960s).[29]

Thus, of the several million Americans who considered themselves overweight in the late 1950s and early 1960s, hundreds of thousands (probably well over a million) of them—mostly women—were fleeced by predatory fat doctors every year. Millions more were medicated, less irresponsibly to be sure, by conventional physicians who were merely conforming to authoritative opinions on reducing weight to fight heart disease, diabetes, and other chronic diseases. As one physician put it in 1955, summarizing his experience treating "369 cases of obese female patients" in Toledo, Ohio, successful weight management rested on the "tripod" of diet, amphetamine, and carefully considered "superficial psychotherapy"—the latter being essential for long-term success. But what doctors like him considered "skill, patience and understanding" may not always have come across as kindness to their fat patients. The Toledo physician reported that among his clients, those who kept regular appointments with him achieved weight loss on average double those who did not. Among this latter group (the bad patients, as it were), there were many "oldtimers" who had already "seen four or five doctors in their efforts to lose weight and who knew every answer"; they were often "markedly neurotic" women with a "heavy load of marital and domestic problems."[30]

Philadelphia doctor Israel Bram, a respected thyroid disease expert who was often consulted about obesity, illustrates another case of a bedside manner that might be considered lacking. During the 1940s, he treated approximately 1,000 fat patients, his approach informed by the dominant psychiatric thinking of the time and his metabolic expertise. One of these patients was "Z," a sixteen-year-old girl who was given "practical psychotherapy," a reducing diet, and "well selected medicaments" (most likely amphetamine and not thyroid hormone, given Bram's view that almost all obesity was "alimentary" and psychosomatic rather than "glandular"). The approach succeeded, in that she lost 50 of her initial 230 pounds in just three months. Seeing her reduction stall and fearing relapse, Bram gave her a pep talk to strengthen her resolve. He followed up with a message that I have trouble imagining a doctor today putting in writing:

> I trust you to carry out the promise you made to cooperate [with the prescribed diet and medication] without question. There are excellent motives for your enthusiastic teamwork. In the first place, you will be safeguarding your future health.

Secondly, of equal importance, is the fact that some day you may want to get married, and we all wish you to be a beautiful bride. Of course, no one wants to be a fat bride, and the time to begin preparing to be a beautiful bride is now. With best wishes and regards, and looking forward to an excellent report from you.[31]

Thus, according to this "practical psychotherapy," fat is the opposite of beautiful. With such condescension and contempt toward fatness even among well-meaning doctors, it is no wonder that mutual aid weight-loss groups, mainly composed of women, tended to keep medicine at a distance.

The Prescription Alternatives for Heart Disease Control

Mainstream physicians wrote diet pill prescriptions in the postwar period because they were concerned about the health consequences of overweight and obesity, and the leading health consequence concerning them was heart disease—especially in men (probably followed by diabetes, at least in women). Getting patients to lose weight was their main option for preventing heart disease because until the end of the 1950s, there was no effective pill that targeted simple high blood pressure (idiopathic or "essential" hypertension, which is high blood pressure associated with no other disease or symptoms) without serious side effects. Patients with very high blood pressure (malignant hypertension) or with hypertension from the kidney disease that often accompanies heart failure were often treated with risky surgery that cut certain sympathetic nerves along the spine. Doctors also prescribed low-salt diets to help the kidneys and sometimes barbiturates, which helped by lowering the heart rate and reducing physical activity. None of these treatments were suitable for active, working adults without any signs or symptoms of heart disease. Physicians eagerly awaited a new medicine they could use more generally in mild hypertension.

There were some false starts that revealed the eagerness doctors felt to intervene against heart disease in ways other than fighting obesity. In 1954, when the drug firm Wyeth put on a show to launch its new Ansolysen hypertension product, a novel chemical with general nerve-blocking effects that reduced blood pressure by expanding peripheral arteries, it "played to capacity houses of MD's in 26 cities via closed TV circuit" and reached a medical audience double the 5,000 expected.[32] However, while Ansolysen proved profitable, the broad and unpleasant side effects of this "ganglionic blocker" drug class—constipation, impotence, and lethargy—limited its usage. Also in the early 1950s, the Indian medicinal herb *Rauwolfia serpentina* was analyzed pharmacologically and tested on heart patients, showing strong blood-pressure-reducing effects. *Rauwolfia* extract and its main active component, reserpine, produced good results when tested on men with essential hypertension, and reserpine was marketed aggressively to reduce blood pressure by the Swiss firm Ciba. Ciba's Serpasil sales boomed in 1954, prompting many competitors to launch their own versions of the unpatentable natural product. But reserpine has strong sedative effects—so strong that psychiatrists adopted it as a "major tranquilizer" for schizophrenic patients in asylums as an alternative to chlorpromazine, the first antipsychotic medication. These mental side effects were of course problematic for the drug's use in general practice to control mildly elevated blood pressure in otherwise normal, busy men (despite efforts to reframe sedation as a beneficial action against mental "tension").[33] Doctors still awaited a magic bullet against blood pressure.

The National Advisory Heart Council, meanwhile, continued to favor biomedical research into the causes of heart disease rather than public health measures. In practice as well as theory, Eisenhower-era advisors saw government's main role as funding the research that, once applied through the initiative of private practitioners and pharmaceutical firms, would in the future improve the population's health. And the PHS did fund heart research, both basic and clinical, especially into fat metabolism and high blood pressure.[34] In 1957 the NIH and the Veterans Administration each launched complex multicenter clinical trials to test various existing blood pressure drugs and combinations, including their effectiveness in cases of mild hypertension.[35] But all the drugs seemed problematic, and progress by the industry was slow, so by early 1958 the NIH was seriously considering establishing a dedicated, federally funded and managed research program in collaboration with pharmaceutical firms to generate and test thousands of chemicals as potential blood pressure medications.[36] As it turned out, the long-anticipated miracle drug for hypertension had just been launched by Merck, obviating the need for such direct market intervention.

In 1956 a Merck research team focused on kidney physiology had discovered a new chemical, chlorothiazide, which boosted salt excretion and looked promising as a new diuretic (a drug used for reducing tissue fluid, not seen then as related to essential hypertension). In the first half of 1957 the new drug, dubbed Diuril, was extensively tested on patients for this purpose using the loose procedures that predominated at the time—mostly impressionistic case studies rather than controlled trials. As historian Jeremy Greene has recounted, when one of the researchers doing a case series publicly announced that the drug was good for hypertension too,

Merck in 1958 hastily repurposed its product as a blood pressure medication rather than a diuretic. Diuril immediately became a blockbuster, in its first year capturing 13 million prescriptions, becoming Merck's top seller and catapulting the firm from thirteenth to fifth place among drug companies in terms of US sales. Ready for an individualistic answer to the heart disease epidemic that was more appealing than weight reduction, doctors prescribed Diuril preventively based on blood pressure numbers alone—often when they were only marginally elevated. The potential market was so obviously huge that Merck's competitors already had copycat diuretic antihypertensives close to introduction by November 1958, and by the mid-1960s Diuril had been superseded among the now enormous class of blood-pressure-reducing agents.[37]

Serum cholesterol had been suspected as a major heart disease risk factor before 1950, which is why some first-generation prospective studies measured it, and the early Framingham results confirmed those suspicions. In 1959 the general public was concerned enough that Ancel and Margaret Keys's cookbook urging their meat- and dairy-minimizing Mediterranean diet for achieving heart health through low cholesterol, *Eat Well and Stay Well*, became a bestseller and went quickly into multiple printings.[38] Private medical practitioners also proved eager to treat heart disease risk by prescribing cholesterol-lowering drugs as soon as they were able. As with hypertension, drug manufacturers anticipated a massive market—tens of millions of patients and billions of dollars annually—for any drug that would lower serum cholesterol without major side effects and therefore retard or possibly even prevent atherosclerosis in people without heart symptoms.

Most cholesterol in the bloodstream comes not from food; it is produced in the liver from other fatty compounds. In mid-1956 a chemist at the small Cincinnati-based Merrell firm discovered a chemical that blocked the cholesterol production pathway. In 1957 the new drug, officially dubbed triparanol and branded MER/29, underwent toxicity testing within the firm on animals, and by 1958 it was distributed for clinical testing on humans to doctors friendly to (and generally paid well by) Merrell. One of them, a professor at the Boston University medical school named William Hollander, was particularly enthusiastic about the new drug, reporting that in his case series the drug had minimal side effects and not only lowered cholesterol, but reduced angina attacks in those suffering this sign of incipient CHD. Most American men should take the drug daily in order to reduce their CHD risk, he thought.[39]

Merrell launched the drug in 1960 with unprecedented fanfare and heavy advertising emphasizing Hollander's results, and physicians responded as the firm hoped. They prescribed it widely to men without signs or symptoms of heart disease or even markedly high cholesterol—for example, the asymptomatic forty-one-year-old father of two Allen Toole, whose doctor told him to take the drug because high cholesterol leads to CHD, so lowering it was in his best interest. In one poll, doctors voted MER/29 "the most important contribution to medical therapy introduced in 1960."[40] The drug proved to be a "Wall Street exciter" too.[41] But after only nine months on the market, reports of hair loss and skin and vision problems began appearing in medical journals. The FDA reopened an investigation of MER/29's safety, and evidence emerged that a fat called desmosterol, which the drug increased by blocking its conversion to cholesterol, had its own harmful effects and that Merrell had been covering up these issues since the first animal tests. In early 1962 Merrell withdrew the drug amid bad publicity, a congressional investigation, and lawsuits—such as that by Allen Toole, who was awarded more than $600,000 in compensation for his permanently blinding cataracts and two years of painful ichthyosis (raw and scaly skin).[42]

The MER/29 fiasco quickly faded from the public eye, overshadowed by another Merrell product, thalidomide, a tranquilizer and morning sickness remedy that was causing serious birth defects in the United States and elsewhere. The double disaster triggered important changes in US drug regulation, which now required companies to submit all toxicity and clinical data to the FDA along with new drug applications. The FDA had finally gained the formal power to judge efficacy along with safety, so that no more drugs lacking proven benefits to outweigh their inevitable side effects and other harms would again come to market.[43] Still, the medical profession remembered MER/29: doctors were wary of routine cholesterol-reducing medications for decades to come. Blood pressure drugs would remain a far more important category until the 1990s, when statins—the generation of anticholesterol agents still in use today—became daily pills for the tens of millions envisaged by Hollander.

Simply because doctors from the late 1950s onward had easy alternatives to reducing patients' weight in order to reduce their risk, managing obesity was bound to decline in importance for preventive medicine, even if obesity's perceived contribution to heart disease had remained the same. But it did not remain the same. While managing heart disease risk by controlling blood pressure rose in popularity among doctors, the perceived importance of obesity as a heart disease driver became less clear, amplifying the decline in obesity's clinical importance.

Fat Kills—But How?

Even without the first generation of reports from Framingham and other prospective epidemiological studies, American cardiologists increasingly accepted the idea that serum cholesterol levels—or, better put, the bloodstream's fat profile—was somehow driving the heart disease epidemic in the United States. Behind this rise in cholesterol's status, which came largely at the expense of obesity, lay the efforts of Ancel Keys and some other epidemiologists to relate heart disease ultimately to dietary fat intake. From this perspective, excess fat consumption was still bad, but not because fatty "rich" foods contained lots of calories and made people overweight—which they did. Rather, eating too much of certain fats caused CHD and also elevated serum cholesterol—a danger sign and possible vehicle of atherosclerosis. Although the rise of the dietary fat model of heart disease and the concomitant decline of obesity as a perceived driver occurred gradually, the shift had major implications for public health approaches to heart disease in the 1960s and 1970s.

The theory rested on two types of evidence. Apart from the epidemiological studies showing that high serum cholesterol correlated with increased CHD risk, there was also a good deal of experimental evidence that when fed to animals, diets rich in saturated fats raised blood cholesterol. There was also evidence that when fed to humans, diets rich in saturated fats raised blood cholesterol and diets rich in unsaturated fats lowered it. There was no direct evidence in animals or humans that diets high in unsaturated and low in saturated fats reduced heart disease rates. That part was inferred from the epidemiology concerning serum cholesterol.[44]

In 1956–1957 an AHA expert committee reviewed all of the available evidence that connected diet to atherosclerosis to assess whether it was strong enough to justify dietary recommendations to reduce heart disease. This idea was a novelty, in that previous dietary recommendations had to do with avoiding nutritional deficiencies—vitamins and minerals—and rested on the harder evidence of experiments showing how much of a nutrient it took to cure deficiency disorders and how too little brought them on.[45] The committee acknowledged the questionable relevance of most of the experimental work relating dietary fat to serum cholesterol, given its basis in naturally vegetarian lab animals, like rabbits, being fed large quantities of animal fats. Nevertheless, the committee found enough consensus to issue the AHA's first set of dietary recommendations. People at particularly high risk of heart disease were told to restrict the proportion of their total calorie intake derived from fat to 25–30 percent and to decrease the proportion of saturated (animal) fats in the fat they did consume. Moreover, they should limit their total calorie intake so as to maintain a normal weight. The committee published a report on the reasoning behind these views in 1957.[46]

Despite the cautious stance and inclusion of weight control in these guidelines, an editorial in the same issue of the AHA's journal *Circulation* undermined the diet-heart message by stressing that "one cannot separate the study of the fats from the total caloric intake" and that overweight and obesity should not be overshadowed by the "present focal point" of cholesterol.[47] Clearly, strong divisions over the relevance of the dietary fat profile remained among the community of heart disease experts. The AHA eventually extended its dietary recommendations to the general public—as opposed to only men at high risk of coronary heart disease (due to hypertension, a bad family history, having suffered a heart attack, and so on)—in 1965.[48]

In the late 1950s, Ancel Keys began planning a multinational prospective study to establish the dietary fat–heart disease connection more convincingly. This ambitious study would involve representative samples of men in seven different countries and use standardized methods for measuring their diets, blood samples, and health outcomes over at least ten years. He found close collaborators in Japan and Finland—developed countries with CHD mortality rates at the extremely low and high ends of the spectrum, respectively—and in four other European countries (Greece, Italy, the Netherlands, and Yugoslavia). His team in Minnesota managed the American arm of what became known as the Seven Countries study. The study began enrolling participants in 1958, starting with Japan. As had Framingham, and based partly on the same constraints, the study targeted smaller cities with hospital facilities and stable populations from which the researchers hoped to recruit the bulk of their local, middle-aged, male inhabitants. Researchers in each country also established samples of two regions with contrasting diets. In this respect, the US arm of the study was an exception, in that it followed the employees of several railroad companies, a choice doubtless driven by convenience (since it was not a true population sample). All told, the study included some 12,000 men between the ages of forty and fifty-nine.[49]

In 1960, a group of researchers affiliated with the AHA and the NHI began planning a much larger, still more rigorous, and direct test of the diet-heart hypothesis through a project called the National Diet-Heart study. With Keys as one of the six lead investigators, the study would randomly assign more than 100,000 American men to different diets and then follow their blood fat profile and health outcomes prospectively over several years. The planners launched a number of pilot projects and feasibility studies, covering such issues as how best to measure cholesterol and other risk factors and how participants' diets could be manipulated. While the preliminary studies worked out well enough, the plan was abandoned, and the full study was never conducted. In part, this was due to expense. But another reason was that the diet-heart theory now seemed to be under adequate investigation by the Seven Countries study, the first five-year results of which would become available in 1969 and 1970.[50]

The initial Seven Countries findings raised the status of serum cholesterol and dietary fat as drivers of CHD. In the initial examinations, blood pressure and cholesterol correlated better with existing heart disease in the volunteers than body weight did. As for new CHD that developed after the participants were inducted into the study, after five years the rates varied across countries in the same way as cardiovascular mortality in the national statistics: Greece and Japan, with their low-fat diets, at the bottom, and the United States and Finland at the top. When the correlation of the main suspects as causes of CHD was examined, the five-year results were iconoclastic in tendency, although not yet strong statistically. High body weight and obesity (which Keys differentiated, insisting on measuring the latter by skinfold thickness rather than weight for height; see chapter 6) both correlated poorly with CHD—but so also did blood pressure, something of an embarrassment that Keys explained away by suggesting that the measuring procedures in the various countries were not as well controlled as the other standardized procedures. More surprisingly, across the countries, heavy smoking appeared to correlate almost inversely with CHD, contrary to most of the earlier American studies, which found smokers to be more prone to heart disease. Keys found this expected correlation among the US participants in his arm of the study, but the clashing evidence from other countries produced confusion about smoking as a direct cause of CHD.[51]

The most important initial outcome of the Seven Countries study was the demonstration that both the serum cholesterol levels of the participants and the proportion of their total diet consisting of saturated fat correlated well with their incidence rates for coronary heart disease. Overall fat consumption did not correlate nearly as well. Diets were more thoroughly assessed than in previous studies: samples of participants were periodically asked to keep careful seven-day diaries of all foods eaten, with each item weighed, and investigators then replicated all reported food items from the diaries and subjected them to a standardized chemical analysis. Interestingly, Keys's Minnesota team did not measure the diet composition of the American participants using the same careful procedures as in the other six countries, so that the correlation between saturated fats and CHD could not be accurately assessed in the United States.[52]

The findings of the Seven Countries study, for all its rigor, were not always statistically significant. Nor were they consistent, in that some correlations found in one country did not exist in others, as with smoking. Somehow, such still-equivocal findings of the diet-heart connection overshadowed alternative causes of CHD, such as obesity, for which there remained strong evidence.[53]

By 1970, the idea that obesity might be a key cause of heart disease was not so much viewed as disproven but seen as unimportant; serum cholesterol, blood pressure, and perhaps smoking overshadowed it. Among doctors and public health authorities, it remained a danger—a factor correlated with the development of CHD, even if many epidemiological studies suggested that obesity was a secondary cause or only indirectly associated via another cause (like blood pressure). Bringing down weight was still supposed to reduce CHD risk. However it was now possible for doctors concerned about heart disease to avoid unrewarding efforts to make fat patients lose weight and instead address other factors by prescribing drugs for blood pressure or by advising the consumption of lower-fat foods—perhaps "Mediterranean" diets. That is partly why obesity became less important. More surprisingly, the idea that Americans were too fat was beginning to fade. Although Americans were on average still getting heavier, a new way of assessing obesity had made it rarer, almost to the point that it was becoming epidemiologically uninteresting. A new definition of obesity had made national fatness all but disappear.

CHAPTER 6

The Disappearance of Obesity as a Public Health Problem

How many Americans were obese, and how important was the answer to the nation's health? The answers to these questions of course depended not just on the population's body measurements and obesity's theorized role in life expectancy, but also on the very definition of obesity. In the mid-1960s, all three of these matters were somewhat uncertain—at least as uncertain as they had been a decade earlier. Researchers disagreed on what effects excess flesh had on people's health. Public health authorities lacked firm information on how many people were obese, by how much, and what the trend was. Physicians had no consensus on what constituted clinical obesity—that is, when a person was fat enough to endanger their health. In fact, there was new confusion about how to even measure obesity.

The 1960s saw public health's constraints of the previous decade lifted to some extent by changes in Washington, DC. John F. Kennedy's New Frontier era brought direct federal intervention to aid the least fortunate Americans, including in the domain of health. His successor as president, Lyndon Baines Johnson, carried the momentum forward with his broad Great Society agenda to share the richest nation's wealth more fairly, including the Medicare program to provide health insurance for most Americans over sixty-five. While public health in the United States maintained its newfound focus on individual behavior to control chronic disease, it echoed the spirit of the age with a new emphasis on disadvantaged groups (whereas obesity was still perceived as a middle-aged, middle-class affliction of middle America). It also began challenging corporate privilege (gingerly, to be sure), most dramatically with the 1964 Surgeon General's Report on Smoking and Health, which officially named cigarette smoking as a health threat—this arguably should have been declared a decade earlier—spawning the field of tobacco control in the Public Health Service's Office of Smoking and Health.[1] Cancer control had a new lease on life, yet the parallel field of obesity control enjoyed no rebirth. Indeed, by the 1970s, obesity was no longer on the PHS's list of foremost health concerns. The science around it had changed.

The American people too had changed. As the many children born during the war and early postwar years entered maturity, the nation became more youthful in its cultural and political orientation. Rebelling against the Cold War siege mentality of their parents and the conformity they perceived in it, the young baby boom generation embraced and experimented with new identities and lifestyles that not long before would have been characterized as deviant and frequently explained in the stigmatizing terms of psychiatric illness. Indeed the sociological study of deviance, from which stigma and labeling theory derive, can be regarded as a scholarly offensive in this generational rebellion.[2] Younger people in the 1960s and 1970s tended to regard the reigning experts' theories about social outsiders—for example, homosexuals, assertive women, and fat people—as repressive instruments of social control, and the views of medical experts were not spared such suspicion.[3] It could be argued that this newly tolerant attitude toward stigmatized groups was part and parcel of the thaw in the Cold War characterizing the era, the period of détente or mutual tolerance between the capitalist West and communist East, in that expert-endorsed stigmatization was an instrument of martial regimentation on the American home front but was now obsolete.

The confluence of these changes in values and the changes in science and in public health's emphases led to obesity becoming uninteresting as a danger, perhaps even unreal. Thus, the end in the 1970s of America's first obesity crisis was multifactorial, to use the language of heart disease epidemiology; it involved shifting social attitudes, politics both within science and without, and interrelated changes in epidemiological knowledge concerning the prevalence of obesity, its contribution to heart disease, and even the seriousness of the heart disease epidemic itself.

Surveying the Nation's Obesity

For more than thirty years, public health authorities had bemoaned their lack of information on the health of Americans. In the 1930s, as I have shown, the desire to learn about health, as well as death, drove public health researchers to survey local populations about their general health conditions and levels of disability. Most of those studies consisted of standardized, brief interviews, which were useful for determining days lost from work due to illness, but not for assessing morbidity as a doctor or epidemiologist would see it. As of the mid-1950s, the best information on the population's physical health still came from the insurance industry, because applicants had to undergo medical examinations to buy life insurance policies—but of course insurance data only described the insurance-purchasing population, which was whiter, wealthier, and healthier than the national population. These data did not fulfill the "needs and desires which have long been felt by American health workers" for a systematic picture of the actual population, based on medical examinations.[4] Nobody actually knew how heavy Americans were, what their blood pressure was like, and so forth.

In 1956, however, the US Congress followed Britain and some other developed countries in funding a series of studies on fully representative samples of the national population, which were designed to assess the country's health in a systematic and standardized way. The explicit purpose for this first National Health Examination Survey (NHES) was to gain better knowledge to guide the distribution of resources in public health and medical research. In the process, the survey would also produce benefits for military planners, the insurance and pharmaceutical industries, and other businesses involved in health. The NHES produced the first true measures of the national prevalence of heart disease and high blood pressure, of weight and height, and of a number of other relevant health characteristics of Americans. It also established the baseline against which subsequent surveys would measure change.[5]

The first cycle of the national survey took place from 1959 to 1962, during which about 6,700 adults were examined (and about four times as many interviewed). The prevalence of high blood pressure in the NHES was similar to that found in the Framingham study—and somewhat alarming. For example, almost one in five men between the ages of forty-five and fifty-four had blood pressure levels high enough (exceeding either 160 mm diastolic or 95 mm systolic) to triple the chance of coronary heart disease, according to the Framingham study's initial findings. Prevalence increased with age, of course, but hypertension was high even among men aged thirty-five to forty-four: one in eight had dangerous hypertension. The picture was considerably worse for African Americans, among whom more than a quarter of similarly aged men suffered from dangerous hypertension.[6]

And if the national blood pressure picture was concerning, the cholesterol findings were terrifying: 20 percent of white men thirty-five to forty-four had serum levels (260 mg/100 ml) that the Framingham researchers linked to a fivefold increase in coronary heart disease over those with low cholesterol. For African Americans, this risk factor was similar. As for CHD itself, the NHES found that about 3 percent of the living adult population had definitely suffered and survived a heart attack. Another 2 percent had signs of advanced coronary disease that foretold an attack. Again, both findings were in line with the observations from Framingham. Of course, since the first sign of CHD is very often a fatal heart attack, the number of people suffering from progressive coronary disease was presumably several times higher.[7]

The survey also found a high prevalence of overweight and obesity, as defined by the standards of the 1950s (which were based on Metropolitan Life's actuarial studies). Comparisons to similar data from Canada and to prior insurance data suggested that Americans were both fatter than their neighbors to the north and fatter than they used to be. American men were, on average, five pounds heavier for their height compared to contemporary Canadians. They were also six to seven pounds heavier than insured (mainly) American men a decade earlier. Women were now six to seven pounds heavier than their Canadian counterparts and ten pounds heavier than insured American women a decade earlier.[8] Looking at these data, even considering the differences in the measurement methods and the groups measured, it was hard to escape the conclusion that Americans had gained weight over the course of the 1950s.

These NHES findings were consistent with Metropolitan's 1951 estimate that at least a quarter of all American adults were overweight, defined then as 10 percent or more above the actuarial "ideal" weight. As for pathological (i.e., medically important) obesity, which Metropolitan had defined as 20 percent or more above ideal weight, fully 25 percent of men thirty-five to forty-four years old met that definition in the NHES survey. The total for all adults was close to 10 percent, double that of Metropolitan's estimate in 1951.[9] That no great furor arose from these findings in the mid-1960s reflects the extent to which both the definition of obesity and its health impact had become more confused than they were a decade earlier.

When the successor survey was done a decade later, its findings showed a continuing trend. The National Health and Nutrition Examination Survey (NHANES 1) conducted in 1970–1972 demonstrated weight gain against the baseline established by the NHES. For example, the median weight of men aged thirty-five to forty-four at the median height of sixty-eight inches had increased from 170 to 174 pounds. Nevertheless, the Public Health Service investigators doing the analysis concluded that a similar—not greater—proportion of the population was overweight in 1970 as in 1960. To reach this conclusion, the researchers used a more stringent standard: now people had to be an extra 5 percent heavier in order to count as overweight. With overweight now defined as 15 percent greater than the ideal weight for a given height—calculating to a BMI of 28 for median men in today's terms, well above the current BMI 25 threshold for overweight—the NHANES 1 concluded that 23 percent of adult men and 29 percent of adult women were overweight to some degree in 1970.[10]

Only the arbitrary change in definition, which the analysts did not justify in terms of health consequences, prevented a more alarming conclusion. Judged on the basis of weight, the proportion of obese Americans by any fixed definition must have markedly increased between 1960 and 1970. But the NHANES 1 report voiced no alarm at the prevalence of obesity in the United States. Its main point, rather, was that true obesity was significantly rarer than Americans' weight suggested and thus that the national fatness problem had been exaggerated: "the proportion of men who were overweight was significantly higher than the proportion of men who were obese"—and the situation was similar for women.[11] The authors derived such seemingly contradictory conclusions from a new way of defining obesity based on levels of fat in the body, as opposed to weight.

The NHANES 1 report defined obesity as "adiposity," or high body fat content, and it was assessed by using calipers to pinch and measure a person's subcutaneous fat thickness in two places. The researchers found that measurements of adiposity made by this skinfold technique did not map directly onto measures of obesity classically defined in terms of weight for height. In place of the Metropolitan tables of ideal weight based on policyholders, the NHANES investigators defined a weight-for-height standard of overweight based on the surveyed population between twenty and twenty-nine years old (consistent with the principle that most people's healthy weight is what they weighed around age twenty-five). At the eighty-fifth weight percentile for twenty- to twenty-nine-year-olds, just half of the 23 percent of the overall male population above that threshold were also excessively fatty—defined as the eighty-fifth percentile of adiposity (measured by skinfold). Half again as many were fatty but not overweight, yielding a "true obesity" prevalence among adult men of 19 percent. Only for the very heftiest people (above the ninety-fifth weight percentile) did the body fat measure produce the same prevalence of obesity as the weight-for-height measure.

It is possible to read the NHANES 1 report as implying that obesity was only a health problem in its extreme form—that is, in the heaviest and fattest 5 percent of the population. In any case, disregarding the insurance studies whose analyses of the contributions of milder overweight to mortality stood undiminished (even if the exact boundaries of actuarial best weight were blurred by measurement with shoes on), the authors wrote that "no critical values of overweight and obesity have been identified at which cardiovascular or other morbidity predictably occur."[12]

That the PHS researchers could say such a thing reflects the degree to which faith in the measurement methods used in the actuarial studies had been eroded. That is, implicitly, Dublin may have conducted elegant analyses, but his underlying numbers were worthless.

The attitude evinced by the NHANES 1 obesity analysts—essentially that half a century of massive insurance studies could be ignored because they were based on bad data about weight and had not measured adiposity—was a common one among epidemiologists in the 1970s. An intricate effort to redefine obesity as high body fat content rather than as excess weight had cast doubt on the proper measurement and prevalence of obesity. The true health risk presented by obesity (defined either way) had, meanwhile, also grown more confusing. The key scientific figure responsible for these changes was Ancel Keys.

Keys and the Conquest of Overweight by BMI

Since the late 1940s, Keys had been at war with the insurance industry's studies showing the correlation of overweight with mortality. He was irritated not only by the industry's measurement methods and what he considered the exaggerated contribution of obesity to heart disease indicated by the insurance studies, but by the very definition of obesity according to weight for height. Thus from the beginning of his own "businessmen" prospective study in 1948, Keys and his collaborators consistently tracked their research subjects' serum cholesterol and body fat content along with weight and height measurements. Keys mainly determined body fat by the thickness of subcutaneous fat measured by pinching the skin in multiple places with calipers, and it was Keys's work along these lines that led to the NHANES 1 adopting the same method of measuring obesity.

At least at first, Keys struggled to produce meaningful information from adiposity measures; neither body fatness nor overweight correlated with CHD among the Minneapolis businessmen. But his small businessmen study was just the start of Keys's efforts to replace the weight-height tables with a new measure of obesity, which he believed would better predict heart disease and better fit his own dietary fat theory. In 1951, a National Research Council (NRC) committee that Keys chaired began a five-year project to evaluate "the nutritional status of man with regard to emaciation, obesity, growth, skeletal and muscular development." The project, led by psychologist Josef Brozek, was based in Keys's physiological hygiene lab at the University of Minnesota. The NRC sponsored the study in part to provide information to the United Nations for its international aid and development activities relating to malnutrition. Under Keys's influence, however, obesity—particularly the quantification of body fat content—became a major focus of the project (even though the United States was the only country in the early postwar world likely to suffer from obesity).[13]

Building on methods that the Keys group had used to measure body fat content during the wartime starvation experiments, Brozek's team developed precision techniques to determine the fatness of their volunteers. The core method involved immersing volunteers underwater in a weighing tank to calculate the body's density. Fat is more buoyant than either bone or muscle mass, so bodies with higher fat content float more easily and therefore show lower specific gravity. Measurements by this method were made more accurate by carefully estimating lung volume by flushing out and capturing all nitrogen exhaled by the research subjects after emptying their lungs. Density calculations were adjusted for variations in specific gravity due to water temperature, of course. The official purpose of all of this elaborate, conspicuously precise obesometric work was to test and calibrate less intrusive measures of fatness, including measurements of subcutaneous fat. Testing many sites on the body and using pinching procedures, the Minnesota researchers ultimately concluded that the most clinically useful measure of body fatness was the sum of the thickness of subcutaneous fat pinched, with a certain level of firmness and a certain design of calipers, just below the scapula and on the back of the upper arm (triceps) held out at ninety degrees. With its endorsement from the NRC, the Keys-Brozek skinfold measure of body fat content was widely adopted among researchers interested in obesity.[14]

Finding a better way to measure body fat content addresses a different question than whether adiposity or weight-height measurement is the better measure of obesity—or whether either is a good predictor of heart disease. Speaking alongside Keys and Brozek at a 1955 conference at which the NRC study results were presented, Herbert Marks of Metropolitan Life Insurance made essentially this point. He defended actuarial mortality studies as a strong basis for predictive correlations between weight-for-height and health outcomes, at least in essentially healthy people (that is, healthier than a national cross-section). Marks recapped the extensive body of insurance industry studies, which showed consistently that people with above-average weights showed excess mortality rates, especially from cardiovascular diseases. Even the insurance industry, he revealed, had explored other body measures as predictors of mortality—for instance, abdominal girth—but actuarial analysis consistently found that weight-for-height most effectively correlated with life expectancy.[15]

Keys encountered additional skepticism from a Public Health Service team also present at the 1955 meeting. Led by Sidney Abraham, who would later participate in the NHANES 1 analysis, the group reported on a multiple screening project that assessed signs of cardiovascular disease, height and weight, and skinfold thickness measured by the recommended Keys-Brozek method. Their study found that among "obese" men, measured in terms of both weight-for-height tables and crude weight, previously unknown heart disease was more than twice as common as among those of average weight-for-height (or simply weight). But the PHS researchers found that skinfold thickness showed no correlation with heart disease: the fatty men and the normal men had statistically equal levels of heart disease.[16]

For the next ten years, Keys attempted to demonstrate not only that dietary fat was a more important cause of heart disease than obesity was, but also that body fat, typically measured by calipers, was a superior index of that risk. For example, the Seven Countries study, with its definitive rigor in assessing the contribution of dietary fat to heart disease, was also designed so that it could show that new heart disease was better predicted by obesity as adiposity defined by skinfold than by obesity as weight for height. When the first Seven Countries findings were released in 1970, Keys argued that obesity measured by skinfold correlated to new coronary heart disease better than did relative weight. He based this conclusion on qualitative impressions, in that the ranking of countries by CHD incidence rate aligned better with the ranking of countries by adiposity than the ranking by overweight.[17] These results, however, were not statistically meaningful.

Keys pressed on. In 1972, he and his collaborators published a more detailed analysis of the Seven Countries study's five-year outcomes, which focused on three different definitions of obesity as predictors of CHD: skinfold adiposity, weight-for height, and BMI (a different weight-height measure calculated as weight in kilograms divided by height in meters squared). Among the American railroad men, relative weight and skinfold thickness each correlated significantly with both "any" and "hard" CHD onset (the latter was a smaller number of cases determined by more rigorous criteria); BMI correlated with neither. Among Northern European (Dutch and Finnish) men, all three measures correlated with "hard" CHD and none with "any." Among Southern European (Italian, Greek, and Yugoslavian) men, on the other hand, BMI correlated with both "hard" and "any" CHD, while skinfolds and relative weight correlated only with "any." (The Japanese men were not analyzed on this aspect.) There was no great advantage to BMI for predicting CHD in this analysis: for the American men it failed compared to the other measures, while for the Southern Europeans it seemed to show a better discrimination of "hard"

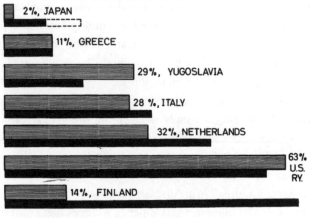

MEN 40-59, % WITH Σ SKINFOLDS > 28 mm

2%, JAPAN

11%, GREECE

29%, YUGOSLAVIA

28 %, ITALY

32%, NETHERLANDS

63% U.S. RY.

14%, FINLAND

NARROW, SOLID BARS SHOW CHD INCIDENCE RATE

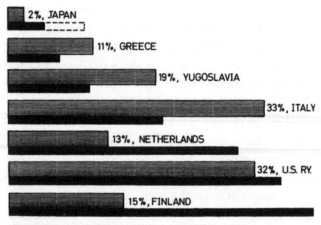

MEN 40-59, % WITH RELATIVE WEIGHT >110 %

2%, JAPAN

11%, GREECE

19%, YUGOSLAVIA

33%, ITALY

13%, NETHERLANDS

32%, U.S. RY.

15%, FINLAND

NARROW, SOLID BARS SHOW CHD INCIDENCE RATE

Ancel Keys argued that obesity as measured by skinfold was qualitatively superior as a predictor of coronary heart disease compared to obesity as measured by relative weight in the Seven Countries study. Reprinted from Ancel Keys and Seven Countries Investigators, "Coronary Heart Disease in Seven Countries: Summary," *Circulation*, suppl., 41, no. S1 (1970): 186–195, figs. S5, S6.

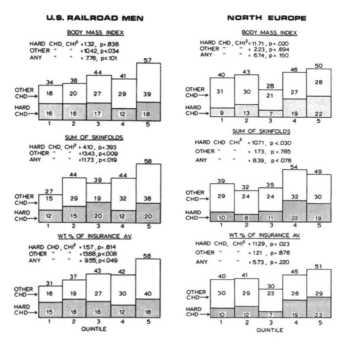

Comparison of three measures of obesity in relation to coronary heart disease (CHD) incidence in American and Northern European men (Seven Countries data at five years). There was no demonstrable superiority of the BMI or skinfold definitions of obesity. Reprinted from Ancel Keys et al., "Coronary Heart Disease: Overweight and Obesity as Risk Factors," *Annals of Internal Medicine* 77, no. 1 (1972): 15–27, figs. 1, 2.

CHD. As for skinfold compared with relative weight, there was no difference whatsoever. Keys ultimately argued that BMI was preferable because it was "easy to calculate, its meaning is unchanging from population to population and from time to time," and it correlates as well as any other measure with body fat content.[18]

So, after twenty years of elaborate and prominent efforts to showcase skinfold and the body fatness it measured as a more rigorously scientific and predictively effective index of obesity, Keys all but dropped the topic of skinfold and adiposity. But his surprising turn away from skinfold is easier to understand if one abandons the premise that Keys's main aim was to clarify the contribution of obesity to heart disease. Perhaps his goal was simply to advance the dietary fat theory of heart disease and to undermine any competing explanations along the way, including obesity defined by overweight. Sowing doubt about the proper definition of obesity was one way to advance that goal; after all, even if it had no better predictive value, replacing weight and height with BMI, on the grounds that it was convenient and

not based on any particular population's weight distribution, had the effect of making insurance studies on obesity's health impact impossible to compare with more
recent studies using the new measure and therefore obsolete. (The technical obstacles to reanalyzing old insurance data in BMI terms were not likely to be sur-
mounted.) Furthermore, by the mid-1970s the diet-heart theory was triumphant
in popular opinion and dominant among experts, even if some harbored reserva-
tions, so it was less important to undercut the alternatives.[19]

By about 1970, Keys's contention that coronary heart disease was probably related to the fat content of the body, as distinct from excessive weight, had gained
much ground in medical thought. This was the case even though Keys's own research on adiposity had not been conclusive on this point. Theories that blamed
body fat rested on indirect evidence, including animal studies, which pointed to
disordered fat metabolism as a driver of CHD. The direct evidence, however, still
showed simply that people with higher serum cholesterol and blood pressure, and
heavier people (often with high cholesterol or high blood pressure) died excessively
from heart disease. The Seven Countries study did not change that picture; it mainly
built the case for dietary saturated fat as a factor raising cholesterol levels.

In any event the activities of one leading scientist are not enough to explain a
major shift in expert thinking and public consciousness about health. In the early
1950s, obesity was thought to be a major threat to people's health; fifteen years later,
public health authorities shrugged. To understand the changing tide of opinions
surrounding obesity's dangers, one must look beyond science to the shifting cultural and political winds that made the voices of skepticism seem more plausible.

The Changing Politics of Fatness in the 1960s and 1970s

As a pathology of excess consumption, obesity was an embarrassment to a
country presenting itself to the world as a consumer's paradise. In the early Cold
War context, obesity suggested there was something deeply wrong with capitalism,
in much the same way as the poor athletic ability of American youth. Under the
Eisenhower administration, the federal government was satisfied for the nation to
address the problem through private initiatives (group weight-loss programs, the
drug industry, fat doctors) and by voluntaristic appeals to national security (the
youth fitness campaign). The leadership of the United States—and the politics of
obesity—underwent a dramatic change in 1961, when forty-three-year-old John F.
Kennedy replaced septuagenarian Dwight Eisenhower in the White House.

Kennedy projected an image of the United States that was dynamic and outward-looking, willing to address its wrongs at home, eager to advance human rights abroad, and prepared to take the initiative to improve the well-being of less fortunate nations everywhere. In keeping with a foreign policy focus on the decolonizing or "developing" world, where a prominent campaign against hunger and poverty was deemed the best way to fight communist influence in Africa and Asia, fighting hunger and injustice at home—especially the problems of African Americans—became a major domestic policy thrust. Obesity in the United States had traditionally been understood as a white problem, a concern of the comfortable majority. As Paul Dudley White put it in a 1962 address, "The United States is the most unhealthy country in the world so far as arteries are concerned; the American diet is the richest"; and the American lifestyle was the most marred by "physical indolence"—making heart disease a special "matter of concern to executives" (like Eisenhower, White's patient).[20] But the public health spotlight was now elsewhere: on improving the lot of the underprivileged.

One of Kennedy's most prominent goals for domestic policy was to achieve what Franklin Roosevelt had not: to establish publicly funded health care for the elderly via Social Security. By the late 1950s it had become apparent even to Eisenhower, whose views in general meshed with those of the American Medical Association, that private health insurance would never meet the needs of poor people and many retirees. In 1956 he signed an amendment to Social Security, which had been passed by a Democratic Congress, that extended monthly payments to disabled workers over fifty. Eisenhower's administration proposed that federal matching grants be provided to states in order to subsidize health care for poor elderly people (if the states chose to provide it), and the proposal became a plank in Richard Nixon's 1960 campaign for president. The counterpart policy plank in Kennedy's campaign provided for hospital care to all elderly Americans, and it was savaged by the AMA. Neither was passed into law, and the Kennedy administration again made federal health insurance for the elderly a key issue in the 1962 midterm elections—again meeting powerful opposition from the AMA and again resulting in a stalemate. But after Kennedy's assassination in November 1963, political opposition to the martyred president's vision slackened. President Lyndon Johnson ultimately succeeded where his predecessors had failed, outmaneuvering Republicans and the AMA with the help of a Democratic surge in the 1964 congressional elections. In 1965 he signed the bill creating Medicare, providing federal insurance for hospital stays and a range of other medical services. It covers all elderly Americans who have paid into it through the Social Security payroll tax mechanism, and while it falls short of a national health insurance plan, it comes closer than anything else in US history.[21]

With the government now responsible for the American population's health more than ever before, one might have expected obesity once again to become a high priority for public health (as cancer prevention through tobacco control did). That it did not reflected the new epidemiological uncertainty around how obesity contributes to heart disease and about what obesity actually is. It also reflected the persistent (and, after the NHES, demonstrably false) image of obesity and heart disease as problems of affluence in a political atmosphere favoring the War on Poverty. But there was, I suggest, an additional reason contributing to disinterest in obesity as a public health problem: the younger generation's suspicion of established experts, especially the type of expert-backed wisdom that located threats to the body politic in the bodies of marginalized classes of people. Civil rights activists fought discriminatory laws and structures, and many who had been previously stigmatized and excluded, including African Americans and other people of color, people with disabilities, gays and lesbians, and even people struggling with drug addiction, gained ground toward full inclusion in American life.[22]

The liberating impulse applied also to the fat. An early manifestation was a 1967 "fat-in" demonstration against discrimination in New York City's Central Park, where about 500 people gathered to burn diet books and destroy an "anti-fat poster" (whether of diet industry or public health origin is unclear). What can loosely be called a fat liberation movement had certainly emerged by 1970, when activist Llewellyn Louderback published an influential book called *Fat Power*. Drawing on his own experience as a large man as well as medical and sociological research, Louderback exposed the diet industry as at best an ineffective swindle and at worst murderous, psychiatry as complicit in harmful stigma, and public health authorities as in thrall to shoddy and inconclusive work by epidemiologists that had failed to demonstrate obesity's harms with any consistency. Louderback also called attention to the many social injustices faced by fat people merely because of their body shape, highlighting prejudices driven by irrational moralism. Soon, courts were deciding employment discrimination cases in line with such arguments.[23]

The vanguard of this early 1970s movement to reinvent social attitudes around fatness—or bigness, as some participants preferred—was the emergence of groups such as the National Association to Aid Fat Americans, Fat Underground, and the Fat Liberation Front, all of which echoed many of Louderback's arguments. They added others too. Fat Underground, for example, declared "doctors are the enemy" and "weight loss is genocide." Ironically, the meetings of these organizations often mirrored the format of the weight-loss groups, including the confessional sharing of humiliating episodes. In this case, though, the aim was not to overcome self-deception so as to accept medical diagnoses of character flaws, but rather to raise consciousness. Participants sought to achieve self-acceptance and political radicalization through recognizing and overcoming such internalized instruments of oppression as the oral fixation diagnosis.[24]

Once a fat activist's consciousness had been raised, the next step was action—specifically, action against medical and commercial weight-loss propaganda. Fat activists spread their liberating countermessage especially to women. While fat women would benefit from their efforts most directly, the activists hoped to bring all women into the fight as "sisters" in their struggle. The thinking and rhetoric matched those of the broader women's health movement in that it critiqued "patriarchal" medicine as pathologizing, colonizing, and managing female bodies. To the fat liberation movement, mainstream medicine was little more than an instrument of oppression and social control.[25]

By 1978 fat liberation fully overlapped with the growing mainstream women's liberation movement, as Susie Orbach's bestselling book *Fat Is a Feminist Issue* attested. Among Orbach's most influential observations was that women are more stigmatized than men for fatness, a claim certainly supported by the advertisements for weight-loss drugs found in medical journals. Orbach argued that women suffer unhealthy body images in part because of men's oppressive expectations and that medical approaches to fat women's bodies involved physical harm and even mutilation—all ideas that radical groups like Fat Underground had been voicing for years.[26]

Evolving Public Health Opinion

In a social environment that was increasingly inhospitable to the old stigmas against fatness, even a mildly stigma-reinforcing public health initiative like that launched by Metropolitan and the PHS against obesity in 1951 ("America's Number One Health Problem") was unimaginable. This popular skepticism about obesity's dangers reinforced efforts among many experts to downgrade obesity as a health threat in favor of dietary saturated fats—that is, Ancel Keys's diet-heart hypothesis. Thus both popular and expert opinions about how big a problem obesity was and what should be done about it evolved under mutual influence in a less alarmist direction from the mid-1960s to the late 1970s, eventually making obesity all but disappear as an officially recognized public health problem.

A good example of expert biomedical opinion on obesity early in this period of change is a 1966 PHS Heart Disease Control Program booklet. Written by public health and nutrition experts, "Obesity and Health" at the outset acknowledged the force of arguments, like Keys's, that distinguished between obesity as high weight for height and obesity as excess body fat. The opening text specifically mentioned that excess body fat was more likely to contribute to illness than mere body weight and that assessments of obesity by relative weight lacked precision compared with fat-measuring techniques such as the skinfold. Indeed, the cover of the booklet featured a skinfold caliper. Still, in what is easily read as a jab at Keys, the authors observed that "concern with technique sometimes overshadows the real purpose for assessing obesity . . . the determination of whether obesity is really a health hazard."[27]

Having dispensed with the caveats, "Obesity and Health" immediately declares that the existing evidence resoundingly supports the conclusion that "a high proportion of our population weighs more than is considered desirable for optimum health."[28] The section discussing obesity levels in the population also takes a conventional line, asserting "a substantial prevalence of obesity at every age in both sexes," based on findings from the insurance industry's Build and Blood Pressure study. The booklet additionally draws on NHES data to note the considerable evidence that Americans had gained weight during the 1950s. Even so, the authors decline to comment on whether obesity, as opposed to overweight, had increased (understandably, since other ways of measuring obesity had been introduced).[29]

The section discussing the health risks from obesity acknowledges Keys's skepticism about the methodological problems in the insurance studies supplying most of the available evidence. However, the booklet includes charts derived from actuarial studies demonstrating the dramatically elevated rates of death from cardiovascular disease and from diabetes correlated even with moderate overweight, but no correlation with most other causes of death. It concludes, "Despite the limitations of the insurance data, the possibility that obesity either directly or by association does cause increased mortality in otherwise healthy people cannot be denied." That is, the preponderance of epidemiological evidence in the mid-1960s still suggested that obesity—even defined conventionally as weight-for-height—contributed to death through coronary heart disease, even if it did not prove that obesity directly caused heart disease.[30] (That the booklet says little about diabetes presumably reflects its origins in the PHS heart disease control program and also the much lower profile of diabetes in national mortality rates.) Therefore, the PHS brochure urges, obesity should be prevented because of the difficulty and danger of weight loss after obesity has already developed.

The section on weight loss likewise is conventional for its day. It adopts the standard assumption that obesity is caused simply by food consumption in excess of needs, and it recommends sensible diets and lightly increased exercise over crash programs, psychological support such as group therapy (mediated by a health professional), and amphetamine for dieters with trouble maintaining their program.[31] "Obesity and Health" backs away from the oral fixation theory of overeating, pointing out that the fat people who consulted psychiatrists were probably unusually disturbed and therefore gave an exaggerated impression of the mental health problems behind obesity. Even so, the PHS booklet endorses the concept of "food addiction" in some fat people, while noting that others may be basically mentally healthy and suffering chiefly from "a conflict with the standards of society." On this score, the booklet devotes considerable attention to the misery caused by overweight due to social stigma. Avoiding this unhappy exclusion was a major reason for obesity prevention.[32]

No comparable PHS publication on the prevalence, dangers, and necessity of controlling obesity seems to have been issued in the 1970s—perhaps significant in itself. The Freudian psychiatry that had underpinned much of obesity control since the Second World War experienced a sharp decline during that decade, in both its influence in medicine and its public credibility.[33] And journalistic exposés and other bad publicity for the diet industry in the late 1960s and early 1970s raised the prospect that the cure for obesity was worse than the condition itself.

These exposés provided shocking details about an arm of the medical profession that seemed more concerned with profits than with protecting patients' health. In January 1968 *Life* magazine's cover had the headline "Dangerous Diet Pills," and the issue included an account by investigative reporter Susanna McBee. Self-described as "slender" and in fact occupying the high margin of her actuarial best weight, she told a story of visiting ten different "fat doctors." All ten of them prescribed and dispensed diet pills to her, even though four of the doctors acknowledged that she was not clinically overweight. By the time she was finished, her medicine cabinet included amphetamines, thyroid hormones, laxatives, and a rainbow of combination tablets. McBee received on average 150 pills from each doctor as a single month's prescription.[34]

The main emphasis of McBee's piece was on bogus fast-buck medicine and the reckless distribution of dangerous drugs. A second theme, however, was how the misery of fat patients made them vulnerable to exploitation. The article began with the tragic story of an "attractive" nineteen-year-old college student, Cheryl Oliver, who appeared only mildly plump as pictured at 160 pounds. Within a year, Oliver was dead after losing 40 pounds through prescription weight-loss pills and strict dieting. At one doctor's practice, McBee was handed a questionnaire that asked, "Do you often feel alone and sad at a party?" and "Do you often wish you were dead?" The gist of the questionnaire and the diet doctor behind it—consistent with the advice in the PHS's 1966 booklet—was that weight loss was essential to escaping social exclusion and misery. "You people aren't going to get down to the weight you should weigh," said a different well-intentioned if hugely condescending fat doctor, who suggested that McBee should just try to lose enough weight to feel happier. These themes were taken up in other major magazines and by two prominent congressional investigations into the weight-loss industry, which contributed strongly to the introduction of tighter regulations on amphetamines in 1971.[35] Obesity control was losing its respectability.

Distinguishing between Obesity as Cause and Obesity as Effect

In the 1970s, epidemiologists continued to question the best way to measure fatness—through skinfolds, relative weight, or BMI. Meanwhile the steady flow of data from the prospective studies solidified their sense that although obesity was in some meaningful way associated with heart disease, high blood pressure and serum cholesterol were more important and more direct causes. A key question now became whether obesity operated as a risk factor in and of itself—that is, as a distinct cause of CHD—or whether obesity was merely the most visible sign of an underlying metabolic disorder (of which high serum cholesterol was probably a more serious manifestation).

As I already noted, the first major set of findings from the Seven Countries study, released in 1970, sowed doubt about the importance of obesity (however defined) in favor of the theory that dietary saturated fat caused CHD by elevating serum cholesterol. These findings resonated with epidemiologists attempting to make sense of the ambiguous twelve-year findings of the Framingham study, released in 1967. The Framingham researchers found no significant correlation between excessive weight for height at initial examination and the study's chief outcome measure, "new CHD"—a composite defined by five different criteria. The Framingham study did, however, demonstrate correlations between obesity, defined as a certain level of excess weight for height above the community median, and two of the conditions included in its definition of new CHD: angina and sudden death (presumed to be due to heart attack). And, in keeping with insurance industry findings, overweight accompanied by hypertension or high cholesterol increased CHD incidence more than each risk factor alone. The overall interpretation was that obesity, even in its milder forms, aggravated existing CHD and precipitated heart attacks, perhaps because excess body weight overworked the heart on exertion, but its independent contribution to CHD mortality was secondary at best.[36]

The sixteen-year Framingham report presented similar data, but the researchers now drew a different conclusion. Whereas the 1967 analysis took a cautious line about obesity as a cause of heart disease, the 1972 report cited this same smooth correlation between heart attacks and degree of overweight as evidence that "obesity appears to contribute to coronary incidence in some unique fashion over and above its association with hypertension," with serum cholesterol, and with other risk factors. This time, the authors explicitly asserted that the "residual effect of adiposity" fully justified efforts to control weight for CHD prevention.[37] Perhaps by 1972 skepticism about the dangers of obesity was so widespread that the Framingham investigators felt a need to defend the value of weight control.

In 1976 the Framingham study's lead investigator, William Kannel, and its statistician, Tavia Gordon, published another analysis specifically pushing back against Keys's downplaying of the risks of obesity as defined by weight. No matter how obesity is measured, they argued, it would still only be an indirect measure of what almost all researchers assumed to be one of the central problems in coronary heart disease: the biochemical consequences of maintaining excess fat tissue. The eighteen years of Framingham data consistently showed that relative weight strongly predicted CHD incidence except at advanced ages and very low weights. The new multivariate analysis, however, made it "evident that much of the effect of obesity is mediated through the other risk factors." Essentially, Kannel and Gordon were suggesting that the *process* of developing obesity—in which the body gains weight by accumulating excess fatty tissue and then maintains that tissue—produced the measured risk factors that epidemiology found to be strongly associated with heart disease. Bodies gaining weight by accumulating fat experience elevated cholesterol, blood pressure, and blood sugar, and these physiological consequences of gaining weight, rather than the excess weight or fatty tissue per se, are what drives coronary disease, they argued.[38]

Kannel and Gordon's argument had important implications for dietary recommendations for preventing heart disease. In the view just described, excess calories, from fat and otherwise, are the ultimate cause of heart disease. Saturated fats are not necessarily dangerous in and of themselves, except to the extent that as a key source of excess calories, they contribute to weight gain. Even slow or minor weight gain above one's ideal weight involves this same pathological process, in line with the insurance studies, and "it can be estimated from Framingham data that if everyone were at optimal weight we would have 25 percent less CHD." In their analysis, therefore, reducing obesity, defined as excess weight, should remain a leading goal of public health: "reduction of overweight is probably the most important hygienic measure (aside from avoidance of cigarettes) available for the control of cardiovascular disease." Contra Keys, they concluded, we cannot "afford iconoclasm while awaiting proof."[39]

This sophisticated analysis by the Framingham statisticians essentially offered a different and partly novel theory of obesity's role in heart disease. The mainstream view—exhibited even in other Framingham publications—considered excess weight, high blood pressure, and high serum cholesterol as independent causes of coronary heart disease. In effect, Kannel and Gordon suggested that all three of these factors were produced by an underlying fattening or obesogenic process that caused heart disease. Although this theory comes close to the expert view of obesity's role in cardiovascular disease in 2018, their view did not catch on in the epidemiological community of their day.[40] Perhaps its distinction from the mainstream notion—that because high cholesterol and high blood pressure were more strongly correlated with CHD, they were more important as causes than overweight—was too subtle. The decline of obesity as a cause of CHD continued in the expert community's estimations.

In the late 1970s, a panel of epidemiologists attempted under AHA auspices to synthesize the proliferating findings from the various prospective studies of CHD into a single authoritative analysis. The Pooling Project incorporated findings from most of the research mentioned in this book, including the civil service studies in Los Angeles and Albany; the Framingham study; Keys's businessmen study and his US component of the Seven Countries study, as well as the results from several other similar first-generation prospective studies not described here. Almost all of the studies demonstrated statistically significant evidence that high blood pressure, high levels of serum cholesterol, and heavy smoking each elevated risk for "major coronary events," such as heart attacks, and new CHD as defined in various other ways. The effects of high relative weight were more modest. When age was factored into the analysis, overweight was a statistically significant risk for men in their forties but not for those in their fifties or older. The Pooling Project's conclusions focused on high serum cholesterol, high blood pressure, and the "pernicious powerful risk factor" of smoking as key causes of CHD, downplaying the risk of obesity.[41]

The ruling epidemiological and medical consensus of the 1970s was that what a person ate was more important to their health than how much—how many calories—they ate. This was the Keys diet-heart view: saturated fats in the diet caused atherosclerosis and therefore heart disease via serum cholesterol. The concept was plausible biologically and epidemiologically. There also existed direct experimental evidence from animals that high levels of saturated fats in the diet could produce atherosclerosis (albeit not heart attacks), while the Seven Countries study showed that saturated fat intake correlated strongly with both serum cholesterol and CHD in humans.[42] Randomized clinical trials involving medications for hypertension showed that lowering blood pressure reduced cardiac morbidity and mortality. (A similar trial involving cholesterol had not been done in the 1960s due to the problems with MER/29, but plans for a trial using a different new drug treatment were in the works.)[43] What had not been tested directly was whether *altering* the saturated fat content of the diet changed the rate of CHD, because the randomized, controlled National Diet-Heart study was never conducted.

It was in this context of strong plausibility that Ancel Keys launched a major study in partnership with cardiologist Ivan Frantz. The Minnesota Coronary Experiment (MCE) was the largest controlled trial of the diet-heart hypothesis ever conducted. One measure of the impressive rigor of this study was that it was double-blind, so that neither subjects nor researchers knew who was receiving what treatment. Between 1968 and 1973, nearly 10,000 patients in six mental hospitals and a nursing home, all in Minnesota, were randomly assigned to either a special diet, which replaced most saturated fats with corn oil (rich in unsaturated fats), or to their regular institutional diet with some corn oil added. Researchers measured serum cholesterol, recorded cardiac events and strokes, and conducted autopsies to assess patients' degree of atherosclerosis and to confirm the numbers of strokes and heart attacks at time of death.

Of the 10,000 original enrollees, roughly 2,400 subjects participated for more than a year, a large enough number to make it a powerful study. But the published results from this research are relatively sparse. Not all the planned analyses seem to have been conducted, and not all those conducted were published. Around the beginning of 1975 Frantz and his collaborators presented some findings at conferences to the effect that the special diets did lower cholesterol. They also indicated that death rates among younger men (but not the other demographic groups) on the low saturated fat diet seemed to decline slightly.[44] The fullest analysis published did not appear until nearly fifteen years later. The delay probably implied to medical audiences that the results were "negative" or not statistically significant and therefore did not merit publication—an ethically problematic but then-conventional practice of medical authorship.[45] As Frantz's 1989 publication eventually put it, cholesterol levels in the experimental groups did drop, but "no differences between the treatment and control groups were observed for cardiovascular events, cardiovascular deaths, or total mortality."[46]

Twenty-first-century scholarship has revealed that behind the scenes, the MCE's results distinctly contradicted the diet-heart hypothesis. Frantz and Keys never published the study's most crucial data: the results from the blinded autopsies. A team of researchers organized by the National Institutes of Health, including Ivan Frantz's son Robert P. Frantz, undertook an elaborate effort to recover and reconstruct these findings. In 2016 this group reported that the overall death rate was actually *higher* among those who received the special unsaturated fat diet, significantly so for subjects over sixty-five. Moreover, reduced levels of serum cholesterol correlated robustly with death rates, again particularly among those over sixty-five. On either diet, those with greater cholesterol reductions died quicker. Finally, many more subjects in the special diet group showed confirmed infarctions compared to the control group, and they also had on average worse atherosclerosis.[47]

This retrospective analysis seems to show that a diet lower in saturated fats conferred no protections against coronary heart disease in the subjects of this study and possibly caused harm. Contrary to the diet-heart hypothesis, neither atherosclerosis nor infarctions, as confirmed by autopsy, correlated with serum cholesterol levels. (These autopsy findings are still considered provisional, however, because only two-thirds of the planned autopsies were ever conducted, and only half of those records were recovered.) One may surmise—indeed, it is now widely suspected—that the study's analysis was stopped and the results not published because they would have shown that lowering serum cholesterol by reducing saturated fats not only failed to reduce mortality from CHD, but was potentially fatal for older people.[48]

What if these "negative" results had been published? Given the size and rigor of the MCE study, as well as Keys's eminence, the publication of its full results might well have undermined or even led to rejection of the diet-heart theory among the medical and public health communities. A similarly designed, large, randomized trial of cholesterol-reducing diets conducted at roughly the same time, the Sydney Diet Heart study, pointed in the same direction but also remained largely unpublished (for reasons having no apparent connection to Keys). Today the data from these two rigorous studies, reanalyzed and combined, are thought to outweigh the published trials supporting the diet-heart hypothesis, and the diet-heart theory is in dispute.[49] While the methods of weighing and combining sets of related trials were in the past less formal, it is reasonable to suppose that if the MCE outcomes had been fully published the diet-heart theory would not have been accepted in the 1970s.

But as it happened, the full results of the MCE and the Sydney Diet Heart study did not see the light of day, and epidemiologists and cardiologists alike embraced the diet-heart hypothesis in the late 1970s. The preponderance of the published evidence, particularly from the Seven Countries study and the Pooling Project (in which Keys also played a lead role), seemed to support it fully.[50] There was no need to worry about obesity when dietary fats seemed a better, more direct explanation of heart disease.

The Politics of Food

By the mid-1970s, the idea that a diet lower in saturated fats was more important to health than weight reduction was almost common knowledge, even though the science was not entirely settled. In 1973, the AHA issued nutrition guidelines that recommended limiting total fat intake to 35 percent of calories (around 10 percent less than standard American meat-and-potatoes diets were said to provide) and saturated fat intake to 10 percent of calories. In 1975 Keys and his wife, Margaret, published a new version of their successful *Eat Well and Stay Well* cookbook called *How to Eat Well and Stay Well the Mediterranean Way*, capitalizing on the cultural currency of the low saturated fat "Mediterranean diet" they had long been promoting. At least a dozen other English-language cookbooks devoted to "Mediterranean" cuisine appeared in the 1970s, three times as many as in the previous decade.[51] Paul Dudley White had written a preface endorsing the original 1959 *Eat Well and Stay Well*, and by now it would be safe to assume that many cardiologists were advising their patients to follow Keys's dietary advice and eat less red meat, eggs, and dairy; use olive oil; and eat more fruits, vegetables, chicken, and seafood. The middle classes in general adopted what one historian has called the "ideology of low fat," and fresh ingredients cooked simply with garlic and olive oil were transubstantiated from peasant food to high cuisine. By the end of the 1970s the ideology spanned all classes, and processed food companies took advantage of the trend with premium lines of "low fat" products for heart health as well as weight loss.

(Soon "low fat" itself became the main selling point, with many successful products containing enough added sugar to offset the reduction in fat calories; the Sugar Research Foundation's strategy was paying off.)[52]

In January 1977, the inevitable resistance from the lobbyists representing adversely affected agricultural industries finally entered the halls of Congress. The controversy involved the Senate Select Committee on Nutrition and Human Needs, which had just issued new dietary guidelines for the United States. In keeping with Keys's and the AHA's recommendations, the new guidelines recommended that Americans reduce their intake of red meat and limit fat consumption to 30 percent of their total calorie intake. Established in the late 1960s to address problems of hunger, this Senate committee had originally been charged with making sure that Americans got enough to eat. By the mid-1970s, however, the committee had turned its attention to the dangers of an unhealthy diet, holding a series of hearings entitled "Diet Related to Killer Diseases." At the first hearing in July 1976, the committee's overall purpose was said to be addressing "the Nation's health crisis" not by federal investment in expensive medical care, but by implementing dietary advice from science to "change our super-rich, fat-loaded, additive and sugar-filled American diet" so as to improve health and longevity, as Republican senator Charles Percy from Illinois put it. While the chair, George McGovern, mentioned obesity's heart dangers repeatedly, a lead witness, Assistant Secretary of Health Theodore Cooper, applauded his concern but redirected the committee's attention to "the role of nutrients, particularly lipids, in the diet" for heart disease. The bulk of that hearing's scientific discussion dealt with cancer and additives.[53]

In February 1977 the committee held two additional days of hearings that focused strictly on obesity, on one hand, and heart disease, on the other, with the goal of establishing what medical experts in these fields thought of the just-released dietary guidelines. The obesity hearing devoted more time to the psychological and social harms of obesity, as well as the problems of weight reduction, than to the confused current evidence on obesity's contribution to heart disease. The expert witnesses by and large agreed that reducing fat in the diet would reduce obesity nationally, and this was treated as a valuable end in itself irrespective of heart disease.[54] In the heart disease hearing, McGovern, prepared better by his staff, this time did not mention obesity in his opening statement. The key expert witnesses were epidemiologist Jeremiah Stamler (a leader in the Pooling Project) and clinical researcher Antonio Gotto, both diet-heart enthusiasts who stressed saturated fats in their testimony, and National Heart, Lung, and Blood Institute director Robert Levy. Gotto explicitly characterized obesity as a "secondary risk factor."[55] Stamler mentioned obesity more, but chiefly as a contributor to high blood pressure. Levy too came across as a believer in the diet-heart theory, agreeing that changing the diet to reduce serum cholesterol would probably save lives and suggesting that, like unsaturated fats, weight loss helped reduce CHD by lowering cholesterol. But he was unwilling to call the theory proven. Diet certainly could lower serum cholesterol, said Levy, but whether lowering cholesterol would actually reduce CHD remained "murky."[56] A conclusive direct intervention to reduce cholesterol in a representative population, and then check the subsequent impact on mortality, had not been tried.

Lobbying groups such as the Meat Board and the Cattlemen's Association, which were worried about beef's "market position," pounced on the hints of scientific controversy that emerged in the researchers' testimony. Under intense pressure, McGovern held further hearings in which the lobbyists' handpicked holdouts against the diet-heart theory aired their doubts: Sir John McMichael, an eminent British cardiologist and outspoken skeptic about epidemiology generally and "the American cholesterol hypothesis" in particular, and the biochemist E. H. Ahrens of the Rockefeller Institute, known for his extraordinarily rigorous standards of evidence (which essentially no epidemiology could meet). Their gist was that, as Levy admitted, nobody had actually shown that lowering serum cholesterol by reducing dietary saturated fats would save lives. The pushback was successful, and in late 1977 the committee issued revised dietary goals that replaced the phrase "reduce consumption of meat" with "choose meats, poultry, and fish which will reduce saturated fat intake."[57]

Several committee staff members resigned in disgust that public health had been subverted to powerful special interests. The mainstream heart disease research community, too, reacted strongly to this episode, closing ranks to defend the diet-heart hypothesis. Several presentations and a plenary lecture at the November 1977 meeting of the AHA reviewed evidence backing the idea that switching to a diet lower in saturated fats reduced serum cholesterol and also (probably) CHD.[58] In 1978 the AHA issued slightly revised diet guidelines that supported the Keys limit of 30 percent of total calories from fat, with a maximum of 10 percent from saturated fats. In 1979 the surgeon general issued a major report called *Healthy People*, which included the "less red meat" recommendation that the Senate committee had ultimately deleted. Once again, meat lobbyists fought back, and this recommendation disappeared in subsequent government publications.[59]

At the same time, scientists critical of the diet-heart theory found themselves treated with intolerance and exclusion, leading Vanderbilt University biochemist

George V. Mann to denounce the mainstream "heart mafia."[60] Thus, given this situation of heightened political tension, the closing of ranks of the mainstream heart disease epidemiology community represents another reason that the diet-heart theory emerged so fully triumphant in the 1970s, eclipsing any remaining worries about obesity as a risk factor and as a public health danger more generally.

In the late 1970s, the problem of heart disease began to seem less urgent. In 1975, Framingham study biostatistician Tavia Gordon published the shocking news that the national mortality rate from coronary heart disease had stopped increasing in the early 1960s; in fact, there was evidence at the time to suggest that it had begun declining.[61] By 1979 this good news was accepted as fact: the heart disease epidemic was receding, and the shift could not be attributed to changes in the way death certificates were completed.

The likely causes for this decline were as complex as the factors that had created the epidemic in the first place. Clinicians had mastered the art of prescribing drugs for hypertension and were presumably recommending diets low in saturated fats more often, in line with the evolving AHA dietary recommendations. Americans were smoking less and possibly exercising more. Improvements in coronary care probably also played a role by extending lives after heart attacks.[62] Furthermore, obesity was apparently leveling out. An analysis of the 1976–1980 NHANES 2 concluded in the mid-1980s that overweight and obesity had not increased in the United States during the 1970s except among black women. Whereas NHANES 1 had found that 23 percent of the adult male population and 29 percent of the adult female population were overweight or obese, defined as the eighty-fifth percentile of weight for height for people in their twenties, NHANES 2 found 24 percent for men and 27 percent for women overall (but 44 percent for black women) by the same definition. Skinfolds were reported, but BMI dominated the analysis, making it hard to compare directly with NHANES 1 except by recalculation; in these terms too there was not much change. For example, the median BMI of men thirty-five to forty-four years old around 1980 actually declined slightly to 25.7, from 26.5 around 1970 (calculated from median height and weight in that age bracket).[63] In 1983 researchers associated with the Framingham study would finally demonstrate with statistical significance that obesity operated as an independent risk factor for new coronary heart disease, albeit half as powerful as high blood pressure and serum cholesterol. But around 1980 the available evidence supported the view that obesity, which appeared to be stable, could not be the main driver behind CHD mortality, which was declining.[64]

When combined with changing notions about the importance of dietary fat as a cause of heart disease, the stabilized prevalence of obesity meant that by the 1980s public health authorities were now justified not to worry about it. While fairly common, obesity was considered dangerous only in extreme degrees. Even if some doubt about the diet-heart theory remained among experts, the idea of an obesity epidemic underlying the heart disease epidemic had died. Few mainstream physicians found obesity interesting, and as amphetamines became stigmatized as addictive drugs in the 1970s and as amphetamine prescriptions became strictly monitored by the Drug Enforcement Administration, doctors steered clear of prescribing diet pills. Instead of hounding stubborn patients to lose weight, they only needed to urge them to watch what kinds of fats they ate or prescribe one of the perpetually new and improved blood pressure medications.[65] For its part, the processed food industry offered an expanding range of tempting "low fat" options to make it easier for dieters to stick to purportedly heart-healthy diets.

The American obesity problem may have plateaued briefly in the 1970s, but despite and perhaps because of this lack of concern, it never really went away. When NHANES 3 was conducted in 1988–1991, it showed that the United States during the 1980s had experienced a substantial increase in overweight and obesity, no matter how it was measured. According to some analyses, levels of obesity and extreme obesity in particular had increased.[66] In the 1990s, public health authorities again raised the alarm about an obesity epidemic, and obesity and its close cognate "metabolic syndrome" were now considered as diseases in themselves. Most twenty-first-century health authorities agree, as they did in the 1950s based on insurance data, that obesity (defined by height and weight according to the current BMI standard) is a strong contributor to cardiovascular disease, kidney disease, and diabetes.

Today, sociologists, epidemiologists, physicians, and fat activists continue to argue over what this new epidemic means, or whether it is a real epidemic at all. Biomedical researchers continue to debate how obesity should be understood and evaluated. While the cultural and political dimensions of the present perceived epidemic are beyond the scope of this book, there are certain resonances with the first epidemic that bear exploration.

Selective attention determines what features of the world scientists measure and what measurements statisticians test for significant correlations. Selective attention made the alarming rise in obesity "the cause" of spiking CHD mortality— "America's Number One Health Problem" in the early 1950s—and made it the epidemic behind the epidemic of heart disease. As I have argued here, that selective attention to obesity was driven by cultural factors like the moralistic view of fatness and softness in the siege mentality of early Cold War popular and political culture. It also owed much to the aspirations of American public health experts during the New Deal and Fair Deal eras, as that profession ambitiously set its sights on expanding from simple hygiene policing and infection control to tackling chronic diseases through case finding, health care provision, and even addressing social determinants of chronic disease, such as poverty. Doctors and medical researchers had additional reasons to focus their attention on obesity in the immediate postwar period. The fashionability of mental health and psychosomatic medicine, the newfound urgency of prevention measures for chronic diseases, and the attraction of new and high-status amphetamine medications all made the obesity epidemic a tempting target for clinical practice. Without access to effective and equally attractive treatments for hypertension and high cholesterol, in the late 1940s and 1950s weight control offered doctors and (more so) public health practitioners the most promising route to reducing heart disease.

Selective attention similarly contributed to the disappearance of the perceived obesity epidemic, even before the decline in CHD was noted. Medical researchers and physicians increasingly turned their focus to dietary fat as a more important cause of heart disease beginning about 1960. Cultural changes such as the destigmatization of fatness; the growing disreputability of the diet industry and its therapeutic mainstay, amphetamine; and the attractive new possibilities for prescribing drugs for high blood pressure and (later) cholesterol all contributed to the waning alarm over obesity.

When historians look back at the discovery—more accurately, the rediscovery—of obesity as a public health crisis in the 1990s, they will almost certainly find the same wide range of factors at play, from culture and politics to the relationships between physicians and the drug industry. How long the present alarm will last, I cannot say, nor do I know what will make it subside. But there is one conclusion I feel certain that future scholars of public health will draw: the health problems associated with the present obesity epidemic were not solved entirely by adjusting individual behavior any more than they were in the first epidemic.

Notes

CHAPTER 1: Fat and the Public's Health before the Second World War

1. Ulrich Beck, *Risk Society: Towards a New Modernity*, trans. Mark Ritter (London: Sage, 1992); Nikolas Rose, "The Politics of Life Itself," *Theory, Culture and Society* 18, no. 6 (2001): 1–30; Adele Clarke et al., "Biomedicalization: Technoscientific Transformations of Health, Illness, and U.S. Biomedicine," *American Sociological Review* 68, no. 2 (2003): 161–194.

2. William Rothstein, *Public Health and the Risk Factor: A History of an Uneven Medical Revolution* (Rochester, NY: University of Rochester Press, 2003); George Rosen, *A History of Public Health* (Baltimore: Johns Hopkins University Press, 2015).

3. For the intersection in public health of "lifestyle" thinking with a biomedical understanding of illness, see Nancy Krieger, *Epidemiology and the People's Health: Theory and Context* (Oxford: Oxford University Press, 2011).

4. Here and elsewhere in the book, when discussing people, I use the term "fat" to refer to the social category as it existed in the early postwar United States. By it, I imply no judgment about people's real health, their appearance, or their actual bodily states. Nor do I deny that there may be health consequences associated with high relative weight—the changing understanding of which is the main topic of this book. My usage of "fat" strictly as a socially defined category accords with how the term is used today in the flourishing field of fat studies. See Esther Rothblum and Sondra Solovay, eds., *The Fat Studies Reader* (New York: New York University Press, 2009).

5. Zoë Harcombe, *The Obesity Epidemic: What Caused It? How Can We Stop It?* (York, England: Columbus Publishing, 2010); Abigail Saguy, *What's Wrong with Fat?* (Oxford: Oxford University Press, 2012); Deborah Lupton, *Fat* (New York: Routledge, 2012); Deborah Cohen, *A Big Fat Crisis: The Hidden Forces behind the Obesity Epidemic and How We Can End It* (New York: Nation Books, 2014).

6. Monte Poen, *Harry S. Truman versus the Medical Lobby: The Genesis of Medicare* (Columbia: University of Missouri Press, 1996), chap. 1; Jaap Kooijman, *. . . And the Pursuit of National Health: The Incremental Strategy toward National Health Insurance in the United States of America* (Atlanta, GA: Rodopi, 1999), chap. 2.

7. Poen, *Harry S. Truman versus the Medical Lobby*, chap. 1; Kooijman, *And the Pursuit of National Health*, chap. 3; Daniel Fox, *Power and Illness: The Failure and Future of American Health Policy* (Berkeley: University of California Press, 1993), chap. 2; Rick Mayes, *Universal Coverage: The Elusive Quest for National Health Insurance* (Ann Arbor: University of Michigan Press, 2004), 34 (quote). On unions, see Alan Derickson, *Health Security for All: Dreams of Universal Health Care in America* (Baltimore: Johns Hopkins University Press, 2005).

8. Poen, *Harry S. Truman versus the Medical Lobby*, chap. 2; Kooijman, *And the Pursuit of National Health*, chap. 3; Michael Grey, *New Deal Medicine: The Rural Health Programs of the Farm Security Administration* (Baltimore: Johns Hopkins University Press, 1999), chap. 6; Harold Maslow, "The Background of the Wagner National Health Bill," *Law and Contemporary Problems* 6, no. 4 (1939): 606–618.

9. Poen, *Harry S. Truman versus the Medical Lobby*, chap. 2; Fox, *Power and Illness*. For an example of public health setbacks in the field of drugs, see Harry Marks, "Revisiting 'the Origins of Compulsory Drug Prescriptions,'" *American Journal of Public Health* 85, no. 1 (1995): 109–115; and Nicolas Rasmussen, "Controlling 'America's Opium': Barbiturate Abuse, Pharmaceutical Regulation, and the Politics of Public Health in the Early Postwar United States," *Journal of Policy History* 29, no. 4 (2017): 543–568.

10. Fox, *Power and Illness*; George Weisz, *Chronic Disease in the Twentieth Century: A History* (Baltimore: Johns Hopkins University Press, 2014), chap. 2.

11. Rosen, *History of Public Health*; Jonathan Liebenau, *Medical Science and Medical Industry: The Formation of the American Pharmaceutical Industry* (New York: Macmillan, 1987); Allan Brandt, *No Magic Bullet: A Social History of Venereal Disease in the United States since 1880* (New York: Oxford University Press, 1987). For an example of an anti-TB initiative involving compulsory reporting, see Arnold Mulder, "Michigan's Part in the War on Tuberculosis," *American Journal of Public Health* 7, no. 2 (1917): 182–186.

12. Arthur Viseltear, "C.-E. A. Winslow and the Early Years of Public Health at Yale, 1915–1925," *Yale Journal of Biology and Medicine* 55 (1982): 137–151; Thomas Parran, "Public Responsibility for Public and Personal Health: The Biggs Health Center Plan of 1920 in Retrospect," *Bulletin of the New York Academy of Medicine* 11, no. 9 (1935): 533–548; Hugh Cumming, "Public Health and the Public Health Service," *California and Western Medicine* 27, no. 1 (1927): 33.

13. Nancy Krieger and Elizabeth Fee, "Measuring Social Inequalities in Health in the United States: A Historical Review, 1900–1950," *International Journal of Health Services* 26, no. 3 (1996): 391–418; Dorothy Porter, "From Social Structure to Social Behaviour in Britain after the Second World War," *Contemporary British History* 16, no. 3 (2002): 58–80; Theodore Brown and Elizabeth Fee, "Henry E. Sigerist: Medical Historian and Social Visionary," *American Journal of Public Health* 93, no. 1 (2003): 60; Theodore Brown, Marcos Cueto, and Elizabeth Fee, "The World Health Organization and the Transition from 'International' to 'Global' Public Health," *American Journal of Public Health* 96, no. 1 (2006): 62–72; Susan Solomon, "The Expert and the State in Russian Public Health: Continuities and Changes across the Revolutionary Divide," in *The History of Public Health and the Modern State*, ed. Dorothy Porter (Amsterdam: Rodopi, 1994), 183–224.

14. C.-E. A. Winslow, "The Untilled Fields of Public Health," *Science* 51 (January 9, 1920): 23–33, quotes 28–29. See also Winslow, "Public Health at the Crossroads," *American Journal of Public Health* 16, no. 11 (1926): 1075–1085.

15. James W. Glover, "Improvement in Mortality Rates and Expectation of Life in the United States from 1890 to 1920," *Science*, n.s., 68, no. 1752 (1928): 73–75.

16. Harold Dorn, "The Increase in Average Length of Life," *Public Health Reports* 52 (1937): 1753–1777.

17. Louis I. Dublin, "The Mortality Trend in the Industrial Population," *American Journal of Public Health* 19, no. 5 (1929): 475–481.

18. Louis I. Dublin, "Memoirs," n.d., folder Memoirs (chaps. 1–10), box 7, 47–63, Louis I. Dublin Papers 1906–1968, MS C 316, Modern Manuscripts Collection, History of Medicine Divi-

sion, US National Library of Medicine, Bethesda, MD (hereafter, Dublin Papers); Herbert Marks, "Body Weight: Facts from Life Insurance Records," *Human Biology* 28, no. 2 (1956): 217–231.

19. Dublin, "Memoirs," chap. 6, Dublin Papers; Dublin, "Can We Extend the Lifespan?," *Harper's Magazine*, May 1930, 766–774; Louis I. Dublin and Mortimer Spiegelman, *The Facts of Life from Birth to Death* (New York: Macmillan, 1951); Isidore Falk, "Louis I. Dublin, November 1, 1882–March 7, 1969," *American Journal of Public Health* 59, no. 7 (1969): 1083–1085; Dan Bouk, *How Our Days Became Numbered: Risk and the Rise of the Statistical Individual* (Chicago: University of Chicago Press, 2015).

20. I. M. Moriyama and Mary Gover, "Statistical Studies of Heart Diseases: I. Heart Diseases and Allied Causes of Death in Relation to Age Changes in the Population," *Public Health Reports* 63, no. 17 (1948): 537–545.

21. Haven Emerson, "Economic Aspects of Heart Disease," *American Heart Journal* 4, no. 3 (1929): 251–267.

22. Bouk, *How Our Days Became Numbered*.

23. Bouk, *How Our Days Became Numbered*; Marks, "Body Weight." See also Association of Life Insurance Medical Directors and Actuarial Society of America, New York, "The Medico-Actuarial Mortality Investigation," vol. 1 (New York: Association of Life Insurance Medical Directors and Actuarial Society of America, 1912); Actuarial Society of America and Association of Life Insurance Medical Directors, "Medical Impairment Study, 1929" (New York: Association of Life Insurance Medical Directors and Actuarial Society of America, 1931); Louis I. Dublin and Herbert Henry Marks, "The Build of Women and Its Relation to Their Mortality," *Proceedings of the Association of Life Insurance Medical Directors of America* 24 (1937): 47–76; Emma Seifrit Weigley, "Average? Ideal? Desirable? A Brief Overview of Height-Weight Tables in the United States," *Journal of the American Dietetic Association* 84, no. 4 (1984): 417–423.

24. This epistemological principle was established in epidemiology well before the pathbreaking postwar studies of cigarette carcinogenicity that are sometimes, incorrectly, credited with its introduction. Richard Doll and A. Bradford Hill, "The Mortality of Doctors in Relation to Their Smoking Habits," *British Medical Journal* 1, no. 4877 (1954): 1451.

25. Louis I. Dublin with Herbert Marks, "The Influence of Weight on Certain Causes of Death," *Human Biology* 2, no. 2 (1930): 159–184.

26. Dorothy Wiehl and Edgar Sydenstricker, "Disabling Sickness in Cotton Mill Communities of South Carolina in 1917: A Study of Sickness Prevalence and Absenteeism, as Recorded in Repeated Canvasses, in Relation to Seasonal Variation, Duration, Sex, Age, and Family Income," *Public Health Reports* 39, no. 24 (1924): 1417–1443, which cites Margaret Loomis Stecker, *Some Recent Morbidity Data* (New York: Metropolitan Life Insurance, 1919).

27. Edgar Sydenstricker, "A Study of Illness in a General Population Group: Hagerstown Morbidity Studies No. I: The Method of Study and General Results," *Public Health Reports* 41, no. 39 (1926): 2069–2088.

28. On Sydenstricker and the economic roots of disease, see Harry Marks, "Epidemiologists Explain Pellagra: Gender, Race, and Political Economy in the Work of Edgar Sydenstricker," *Journal of the History of Medicine and Allied Sciences* 58, no. 1 (2003): 34–55.

29. S. D. Collins, "Causes of Illness in 9,000 Families, Based on Nation-Wide Periodic Canvasses, 1928–1931," *Public Health Reports* 48, no. 12 (1933): 283–308.

30. I. S. Falk, "The Committee on the Costs of Medical Care—25 Years of Progress: I. Introductory Remarks," *American Journal of Public Health* 48, no. 8 (1958): 979–982; Dublin, "Memoirs," n.d., folder Memoirs (chaps. 11–20), box 21, 166, Dublin Papers. Only around the year 2000

did the majority of American physicians come to support universal care with public funding; see Ronald Ackermann and Aaron E. Carroll, "Support for National Health Insurance among US Physicians: A National Survey," *Annals of Internal Medicine* 139, no. 10 (2003): 795–801.

31. P. S. Lawrence, "Chronic Illness and Socioeconomic Status," *Public Health Reports* 63, no. 47 (1948): 1507–1521. Also see George St. J. Perrott and Selwyn Collins, "Relation of Sickness to Income and Income Change in 10 Surveyed Communities: Health and Depression Studies No. 1: Method of Study and General Results for Each Locality," *Public Health Reports* 50, no. 18 (1935): 595–622; George Weisz, "Epidemiology and Health Care Reform: The National Health Survey of 1935–1936," *American Journal of Public Health* 101, no. 3 (2011): 438–447.

32. Weisz, *Chronic Disease in the Twentieth Century*, chap. 4.

33. George St. J. Perrott, Clark Tibbitts, and Rollo Britten, "The National Health Survey: Scope and Method of the Nation-Wide Canvass of Sickness in Relation to Its Social and Economic Setting," *Public Health Reports* 54, no. 37 (1939): 1663–1687; Weisz, "Epidemiology and Health Care Reform," 438–447.

34. Rollo Britten, Selwyn Collins, and James Fitzgerald, "The National Health Survey: Some General Findings as to Disease, Accidents, and Impairments in Urban Areas," *Public Health Reports* 55, no. 11 (1940): 444–470; Weisz, "Epidemiology and Health Care Reform," 438–447.

35. Antonio Ciocco, "Chronic Sickness in Relation to Survivorship Twenty Years Later," *Human Biology* 18, no. 1 (1946): 33–48; Lawrence, "Chronic Illness," 1507–1521.

36. A. M. Master, H. L. Jaffe, and S. Dack, "The Prevalence of Coronary Artery Occlusion," *New York State Journal of Medicine* 39 (October 1939): 1937; Louis I. Dublin, "Heart Disease and Public Health: Current Trends and Prospects," *American Heart Journal* 23, no. 1 (1942): 16–21; Weisz, *Chronic Disease in the Twentieth Century*.

37. Howard Sprague and Paul Dudley White, "The Etiology of Heart Disease with Special Reference to the Present Status of the Prevention of Heart Disease," *Journal of the American Medical Association* 105, no. 18 (1935): 1391–1394; Richard Harrison Shryock, *National Tuberculosis Association, 1904–1954: A Study of the Voluntary Health Movement in the United States* (New York: National Tuberculosis Association, 1957); Daniel J. Wilson, "Basil O'Connor, the National Foundation for Infantile Paralysis and the Reorganization of Polio Research in the United, 1935–41," *Journal of the History of Medicine and Allied Sciences* 70, no. 3 (2015): 394–424; "Voluntary Health Agencies," 1944, folder 10, box 105, file PSF General, Truman Papers, Truman Library, Independence, MO; Bruce Fye, *American Cardiology: The History of a Specialty and Its College* (Baltimore: Johns Hopkins University Press, 1996). The NCI budget in 1943 was $535,000; see "History of Congressional Appropriations, 1938–1949," National Institutes of Health, https://officeofbudget .od.nih.gov/approp_hist.html.

38. James Patterson, *The Dread Disease: Cancer and Modern American Culture* (Cambridge, MA: Harvard University Press, 1987), chap. 5; Victoria Harden, *Inventing the NIH: Federal Biomedical Research Policy, 1887–1937* (Baltimore: Johns Hopkins University Press, 1986); Ronald Hamowy, *Government and Public Health in America* (Cheltenham, England: Edward Elgar, 2007), chap 4.

CHAPTER 2: Obesity Becomes a Mental Disorder

1. Gerald N. Grob, "Creation of the National Institute of Mental Health," *Public Health Reports* 111, no. 4 (1996): 378–381; Albert Deutsch, *The Shame of the States* (New York: Harcourt Brace, 1948); Elaine Tyler May, *Homeward Bound: American Families in the Cold War Era* (New York:

Basic Books, 1988); Nathan Hale Jr., *The Rise and Crisis of Psychoanalysis in the United States: Freud and the Americans, 1917–1985* (New York: Oxford University Press, 1995); Jonathan Metzl, *Prozac on the Couch: Prescribing Gender in the Era of Wonder Drugs* (Durham, NC: Duke University Press, 2003); Alan Petigny, *The Permissive Society: America, 1941–1965* (New York: Cambridge University Press 2009); Ian Dowbiggin, *The Quest for Mental Health: A Tale of Science, Medicine, Scandal, Sorrow, and Mass Society* (Cambridge: Cambridge University Press, 2011).

2. Merriley Borell, "Brown Sequard's Organotherapy and Its Appearance in America at the End of the Nineteenth Century," *Bulletin of the History of Medicine* 50, no. 3 (1976): 309–320; David Hamilton, *The Monkey Gland Affair* (London: Chatto and Windus, 1986).

3. On Adrenalin, see John Parascandola, *The Development of American Pharmacology: John J. Abel and the Shaping of a Discipline* (Baltimore: Johns Hopkins University Press, 1992). See also Michael Bliss, *The Discovery of Insulin* (Chicago: University of Chicago Press, 1982); V. C. Medvei, *The History of Clinical Endocrinology: A Comprehensive Account of Endocrinology from Earliest Times to the Present Day* (Pearl River, NY: Parthenon, 1993); Nelly Oudshoorn, *Beyond the Natural Body: An Archaeology of Sex Hormones* (London: Routledge, 1994). On Kendall, see Edward C. Kendall, *Thyroxine* (New York: American Chemical Society, 1929); Nicolas Rasmussen, "The Moral Economy of the Drug Company–Medical Scientist Collaboration in Interwar America," *Social Studies of Science* 34, no. 2 (2004): 161–185.

4. The "gold rush" term was used by endocrinologist Robert Frank, *The Female Sex Hormone* (Baltimore: Charles C Thomas, 1929), and quoted by Oudshoorn, *Beyond the Natural Body*, 88.

5. Hans Lisser, "The Frequency of Endogenous Endocrine Obesity and Its Treatment by Glandular Therapy," *California and Western Medicine* 22, no. 10 (1924): 509–513, quotes 510. For a brief account of the thyroid-pituitary connection's history, see Patricia Joseph-Bravo et al., "60 Years of Neuroendocrinology: TRH, the First Hypophysiotropic Releasing Hormone Isolated: Control of the Pituitary-Thyroid Axis," *Journal of Endocrinology* 226, no. 2 (2015): T85–T100.

6. W. A. Evans, "How to Keep Well: Study in Ductless Gland Types," *Chicago Tribune*, January 14, 1927, 10.

7. Laura Dawes, "Husky Dick and Chubby Jane: A Century of Childhood Obesity in the United States," PhD diss., Harvard University, 2010, 242; Lewellys F. Barker, "The Obesities: Their Origins and Some of the Methods of Reducing Them," *California and Western Medicine* 37, no. 2 (1932): 73–81.

8. Hans Lisser, "The Endocrine Society: The First Forty Years (1917–1957)," *Endocrinology* 80, no. 1 (1967): 5–28, quote 6.

9. Amanda M. Czerniawski, "From Average to Ideal: The Evolution of the Height and Weight Table in the United States, 1836–1943," *Social Science History* 31, no. 2 (2007): 273–296.

10. Lisser, "Frequency of Endogenous Endocrine Obesity."

11. Lisser, "Frequency of Endogenous Endocrine Obesity," 510.

12. "Personal to Fat Girls" (Marmola advertisement), *San Bernardino Sun*, May 14, 1937, 6; "Men Avoided Me" (Marmola advertisement), *Woman's World*, July 1937, 26.

13. "Heiress' Death Is Charged to Anti-fat Pills," *Chicago Tribune*, September 15, 1937, 1; "F.T.C. Curbs Maker of Reducing Drug," *New York Times*, January 25, 1937, 21; Lesley Fair, "FTC Milestones: Weighing in on Weight Loss Cases," *Federal Trade Commission*, last modified December 4, 2014, https://www.ftc.gov/news-events/blogs/competition-matters/2014/12/ftc-milestones-weighing-weight-loss-cases; John P. Swann, "FDA and the Practice of Pharmacy: Prescription Drug Regulation before the Durham-Humphrey Amendment of 1951," *Pharmacy in History* 36, no. 2 (1994): 55–70.

14. L. H. Newburgh and Margaret Woodwell Johnston, "The Nature of Obesity," *Journal of Clinical Investigation* 8, no. 2 (1930): 197–213; Newburgh, "The Cause of Obesity," *Journal of the American Medical Association* 97, no. 23 (1931): 1659–1663; Newburgh, "The Importance of Actually Measuring the Total Heat Production," *Annals of Internal Medicine* 8, no. 4 (1934): 459–467; Newburgh, "Obesity," *Archives of Internal Medicine* 70, no. 6 (1942): 1033–1096.

15. Newburgh and Johnston, "Nature of Obesity," 211–212.

16. "Just Gluttony Makes Obesity," *Los Angeles Times*, January 5, 1932, 3.

17. Hillel Schwartz, *Never Satisfied: A Cultural History of Diets, Fantasies, and Fat* (New York: Free Press, 1986); Peter Stearns, *Fat History: Bodies and Beauty in the Modern West* (New York: New York University Press, 2002); Sander Gilman, *Fat: A Cultural History of Obesity* (New York: Polity, 2008).

18. Stearns, *Fat History*; Annemarie Jutel, "Does Size Really Matter? Weight and Values in Public Health," *Perspectives in Biology and Medicine* 44, no. 2 (2001): 283–296.

19. "Fat Is Still Taboo, but Chic Frocks Call for Curves," *Chicago Tribune*, May 22, 1929, 40; "1929 Belles Are Not Fat," *Baltimore Sun*, January 27, 1929, 61.

20. Lisser, "Frequency of Endogenous Endocrine Obesity," 510; Lois Banner, *American Beauty* (New York: Knopf, 1983); Stearns, *Fat History*; Gilman, *Fat*; Jutel, "Does Size Really Matter?," 283–296; Amy Erdman Farrell, *Fat Shame: Stigma and the Fat Body in American Culture* (New York: New York University Press, 2011), chap 4.

21. Antoinette Donnelly, "Why Be a Stodgy Fat Vegetable When You Can Be a Flower?," *Chicago Tribune*, October 15, 1927, 16.

22. "Expert Issues Gland Warning," *Los Angeles Times*, May 26, 1930, A12; "Turn to Glands as Key to Hope of Perfect Race," *Chicago Tribune*, January 25, 1931, 25; "Fat Blamed Entirely on Over-Eating," *Los Angeles Times*, June 12, 1931, 1; "Just Gluttony Makes Obesity," 3.

23. Ida Jean Kain, "Overweights Prefer Obesity to Cure—Diet," *Washington Post*, February 26, 1940, 11; Kain, "Overweights' Alibi of 'Glands' Seldom Has Basis in Fact," *Washington Post*, November 25, 1940, 11; Logan Clendening, "Overweight Causes Same in Young, Old," *Washington Post*, June 22, 1940, 11.

24. Joanne Hutch Bruch, *Unlocking the Golden Cage: An Intimate Biography of Hilde Bruch, M.D.* (Carlsbad, CA: Gürze, 1996); Dawes, "Husky Dick and Chubby Jane," 300–356; Miriam Kass, "Dr. Hilde Bruch, Psychoanalyst, Professor, Author, and World Renowned Expert on Obesity," *Houston Post*, August 24, 1973, 2–3AA.

25. Jane Preston and Hannah Decker, "APA Interviews of Hilde Bruch (Transcript)," 1974, 1975, Hilde Bruch Papers, Texas Medical Center Archive, Houston, quoted in Dawes, "Husky Dick and Chubby Jane," 318; Kass, "Dr. Hilde Bruch," 3AA. On the chairs, see Hilde Bruch, "Obesity in Childhood: IV. Energy Expenditure of Obese Children," *American Journal of Diseases of Children* 60, no. 5 (1940): 1082–1109.

26. Hilde Bruch, "Obesity in Childhood: I. Physical Growth and Development of Obese Children," *American Journal of Diseases of Children* 58, no. 3 (1939): 457–484. For a talk describing the six-year-old and his treatment with "follutein" (she does not specify if the hormone was pituitary or chorionic in source), see Bruch, "Obesity in Children," October 1939, folder 1, box 1, ser. III, Hilde Bruch Papers, John P. McGovern Historical Collections, Houston Academy of Medicine, Texas Medical Center Library, Houston.

27. Hilde Bruch, "Obesity in Childhood: II. Basal Metabolism and Serum Cholesterol of Obese Children," *American Journal of Diseases of Children* 58, no. 5 (1939): 1001–1022; Fritz B. Talbot, Edwin B. Wilson, and Jane Worcester, "Basal Metabolism of Girls: Physiologic Back-

ground and Application of Standards," *American Journal of Diseases of Children* 53, no. 1 (1937): 273–347.

28. Hilde Bruch, "Obesity in Childhood: IV. Energy Expenditure of Obese Children," *American Journal of Diseases of Children* 60, no. 5 (1940): 1082–1109.

29. Hilde Bruch, "Obesity in Childhood: III. Physiologic and Psychologic Aspects of the Food Intake of Obese Children," *American Journal of Diseases of Children* 59, no. 4 (1940): 739–781.

30. Hilde Bruch and Grace Touraine, "Obesity in Childhood: V. The Family Frame of Obese Children," *Psychosomatic Medicine* 2, no. 2 (1940): 141–206, quotes 153.

31. Bruch and Touraine, "Obesity in Childhood: V," 175.

32. Hilde Bruch, "Obesity in Childhood and Personality Developments," *American Journal of Orthopedics* 11, no. 3 (1941): 467–474, 473.

33. Dawes, "Husky Dick and Chubby Jane," 314.

34. Bruch fellowship acceptance form, January 1941, folder 119, box 5, Record Group RF 200E, Rockefeller Archive Center, Sleepy Hollow, NY. For background, see E. G. Witenberg, "Janet Rioch Bard, 1905–1974," *Psychiatry* 38, no. 2 (1975): 205–206; Robert C. Powell, "Helen Flanders Dunbar (1902–1959) and a Holistic Approach to Psychosomatic Problems: I. The Rise and Fall of a Medical Philosophy," *Psychiatric Quarterly* 49, no. 2 (1977): 133–152; Hale, *Rise and Crisis of Psychoanalysis*, 167–184; Helen Swick Perry, *Psychiatrist of America: The Life of Harry Stack Sullivan* (Cambridge, MA: Belknap Press, 1982); Dawes, "Husky Dick and Chubby Jane," 325–327.

35. Hale, *Rise and Crisis of Psychoanalysis*; Ellen Herman, *The Romance of American Psychology: Political Culture in the Age of Experts* (Berkeley: University of California Press, 1995).

36. For examples of psychoanalytic "confirmation" of Bruch's oral fixation account of obesity, see A. Rascovsky, M. W. de Rascovsky, and T. Schlossberg, "Basic Psychic Structure of the Obese," *International Journal of Psychoanalysis* 31 (1950): 144–149; Arthur P. Burdon and Louis Paul, "Obesity: A Review of the Literature, Stressing the Psychosomatic Approach," *Psychiatric Quarterly* 25, no. 1 (1951): 568–580.

37. An especially clear psychoanalytic precedent, not cited by Reeve, was Mosche Wulff, "Über einen interessanten oralen Symptomenkomplex und seine Beziehung zur Sucht: Vortrag in der Deutschen Psychoanalytischen Gese," *Internationale Zeitschrift für Psychoanalyse* 18, no. 3 (1932): 281–302.

38. G. H. Reeve, "Psychological Factors in Obesity," *American Journal of Orthopedics* 12, no. 4 (1942): 674–678.

39. Henry B. Richardson, "Obesity and Neurosis," *Psychiatric Quarterly* 20, no. 3 (1945): 400–424, quotes 410, 422; also see Richardson, "Obesity as a Manifestation of Neurosis," *Medical Clinics of North America* 30 (1946): 1187–1202.

40. Otto Fenichel, *The Psychoanalytic Theory of Neurosis* (1945; repr., London: Routledge, 1996), 346–352, 297 (perversion classification). On "narcotics" and addiction in the United States, see David F. Musto, *The American Disease: Origins of Narcotic Control* (New York: Oxford University Press, 1999); Caroline Jean Acker, *Creating the American Junkie: Addiction Research in the Classic Era of Narcotic Control* (Baltimore: Johns Hopkins University Press, 2002); Nancy Campbell, *Discovering Addiction: The Science and Politics of Substance Abuse Research* (Ann Arbor: University of Michigan Press, 2002). One could argue that the mid-twentieth-century American junkie is the paradigmatic "deviant" and "spoiled identity" that defines the stigma concept as deployed by subsequent sociology. See Howard Becker, *Outsiders: Studies in the Sociology of Deviance* (New York: Free Press, 1963); Erving Goffman, *Stigma: Notes on the Management of Spoiled Identity* (New York: Simon and Schuster, 1963).

41. Fenichel, *Psychoanalytic Theory of Neurosis*, 219–220.

42. Gustav Bychowski, "On Neurotic Obesity," *Psychoanalytic Review* 37, no. 4 (1950): 301–319, quote 318.

43. Israel Bram, "Psychic Factors in Obesity: Observation in over 1,000 Cases," *Archives of Pediatrics* 67, no. 12 (1950): 543–552, quotes 543.

44. David Riesman, *The Lonely Crowd: A Study of the Changing American Character* (New Haven, CT: Yale University Press, 1950), 150.

45. Herman, *Romance of American Psychology*; Ben Shephard, *A War of Nerves: Soldiers and Psychiatrists, 1914–1994* (London: Jonathan Cape, 2000).

46. Grob, "Creation of the National Institute of Mental Health"; Gerald N. Grob, "The Forging of Mental Health Policy in America: World War II to New Frontier," *Journal of the History of Medicine and Allied Sciences* 42, no. 4 (1987): 410–446.

47. Statement of Charles Schlaifer, Health Inquiry Hearings, House Committee on Interstate and Foreign Commerce [Subcommittee on Health], [re H-1420-5-D], 83rd Cong., 1st sess., October 8, 1953, 1050.

48. Metzl, *Prozac on the Couch*; Nicolas Rasmussen, *On Speed: The Many Lives of Amphetamine* (New York: New York University Press, 2008); Andrea Tone, *The Age of Anxiety: A History of America's Turbulent Affair with Tranquilizers* (New York: Basic Books, 2008); David Herzberg, *Happy Pills in America: From Miltown to Prozac* (Baltimore: Johns Hopkins University Press, 2009). The Broadway tune is "Gee, Officer Krupke" (lyrics by Stephen Sondheim, music by Leonard Bernstein).

49. Petigny, *Permissive Society*; May, *Homeward Bound*.

50. William L. Laurence, "Psychological Disorders Called the Primary Cause of Obesity," *New York Times*, October 8, 1947, 27; "Fear Keeps Some People Fat, Columbia U. Doctor Says," *Washington Post*, October 8, 1947, 12; "If You're Too Plump, Girls, Stop Being Afraid of Men," *Los Angeles Times*, May 10, 1947, D20.

51. Robert H. Williams et al., "Obesity and Its Treatment, with Particular Reference to the Use of Anorexigenic Compounds," *Annals of Internal Medicine* 29, no. 3 (1948): 510–532; M. B. Hecht, "Obesity in Women: A Psychiatric Study," *Psychiatric Quarterly* 29, no. 2 (1955): 203–231.

52. Walter W. Hamburger, "Emotional Aspects of Obesity," *Medical Clinics of North America* 35, no. 2 (1951): 483–499.

53. Albert Stunkard, "Physical Activity, Emotions, and Human Obesity," *Psychosomatic Medicine* 20, no. 5 (1958): 366–372; Stunkard, "Eating Patterns and Obesity," *Psychiatric Quarterly* 33, no. 2 (1959): 284–295.

54. Opinion of Judge Biggs, *Smith, Kline & French Laboratories v. Clark & Clark et al.*, 157 F. 2d 725 (3rd Cir. 1946); Opinion of Judge Forman, *SKF v. Clark & Clark*, 62 F. Supp. 971 (NJ 1945).

55. Rasmussen, *On Speed*, chaps. 1–2.

56. Mark Lesses and Abraham Myerson, "Human Autonomic Pharmacology: XVI. Benzedrine Sulfate as an Aid in the Treatment of Obesity," *New England Journal of Medicine* 218 (1938): 119–124; Nicolas Rasmussen, "Making the First Anti-depressant: Amphetamine in American Medicine, 1929–1950," *Journal of the History of Medicine and Allied Sciences* 61, no. 3 (2006): 288–323.

57. S. C. Harris, A. C. Ivy, and L. M. Searle, "The Mechanism of Amphetamine-Induced Loss of Weight: A Consideration of the Theory of Hunger and Appetite," *Journal of the American Medical Association* 134, no. 17 (1947): 1468–1475. See also Council on Pharmacy and Chemistry, "Drugs for Obesity," *Journal of the American Medical Association* 134, no. 6 (1947): 527–529; Rasmussen, *On Speed*, chap. 4.

58. "For Medically Sound Reduction of Overweight" (Benzedrine advertisement), *Minnesota Medicine* 31, no. 3 (1948): 317; "For Medically Sound Reduction of Overweight" (Benzedrine advertisement), *Journal of the American Medical Association* 141, no. 12 (1949): 13. See also "Benzedrine . . . for Use in Control of Obesity Has Been Accepted by the Council on Pharmacy of the American Medical Association," *Journal of the American Medical Association* 133, no. 1 (1947): 30–31.

59. "The Happy Fat Man: A Popular Misconception" (Benzedrine advertisement), *Journal of the American Medical Association* 145, no. 7 (1951): 75; "For the Unhappy Fat Man" (Benzedrine advertisement), *Journal of the American Medical Association* 147, no. 7 (1951): 18; "For Centuries, Fat People Were Considered Jolly People" (Benzedrine advertisement), *Journal of the American Medical Association* 149, no. 2 (1952): n.p.

60. "Depression and Obesity Often Go Hand in Hand" (Dexedrine spansule advertisement), *Journal of the American Medical Association* 159, no. 18 (1955): n.p. There may have been earlier advertisements with an addiction theme; medical libraries routinely cut the advertising pages when they bind journals, so few of the ads survive.

61. "Overcoming Weight Control Obstacles" (Obedrin advertisement), *California Medicine* 80, no. 6 (1954): n.p.

62. Clearly the judgment-deflecting "sick role" identified by sociologists in this period had its limits, at least for mental conditions. T. Parsons, "Illness and the Role of the Physician: A Sociological Perspective," *American Journal of Orthopedics* 21, no. 3 (1951): 452–460. For a view on addiction in late nineteenth-century Britain that is similar to mine regarding obesity in the United States, see Virginia Berridge, "Morality and Medical Science: Concepts of Narcotic Addiction in Britain, 1820–1926," *Annals of Science* 36, no. 1 (1979): 67–85.

63. James Gilbert, *A Cycle of Outrage: America's Reaction to the Juvenile Delinquent in the 1950s* (Oxford: Oxford University Press, 1988); Ellen Schrecker, *Many Are the Crimes: McCarthyism in America* (Princeton, NJ: Princeton University Press, 1999); Acker, *Creating the American Junkie*; David K. Johnson, *The Lavender Scare: The Cold War Persecution of Gays and Lesbians in the Federal Government* (Chicago: University of Chicago Press, 2009).

64. This tactic increasingly became characteristic of late twentieth-century public health. See Alan Petersen and Deborah Lupton, *The New Public Health: Health and Self in the Age of Risk* (London: Sage, 1996); Eve Kosofsky Sedgwick, *Tendencies* (Durham, NC: Duke University Press, 1993), 130–145.

CHAPTER 3: The Postwar Heart Alarm

1. Bruce Fye, *American Cardiology: The History of a Specialty and Its College* (Baltimore: Johns Hopkins University Press, 1996), chap. 3; "Heart Week Drive Will Open Today," *New York Times*, February 8, 1948, 5; Roy Gibbons, "Funds Can Cut Heart Disease Toll, 200 Told," *Chicago Tribune*, February 11, 1948, 27; "Record of Correspondence concerning Charles Connor," January 25, 1948, folder 1, box 575, file OF 103, Truman Papers, Truman Library, Independence, MO (hereafter, Truman Papers). See the Truman statement of February 7, 1948, in Office of the Federal Register, *Public Papers of the Presidents of the United States, Containing the Public Messages, Speeches, and Statements of the President, January 1 to December 31, 1948* (Washington, DC: Government Printing Office, 1964), 130.

2. Elaine Tyler May, *Homeward Bound: American Families in the Cold War Era*, rev. ed. (New York: Basic Books, 2008); Eva Moskowitz, *In Therapy We Trust: America's Obsession with Self-*

Fulfillment (Baltimore: Johns Hopkins University Press, 2001); Alan Petigny, *The Permissive Society: America, 1941–1965* (New York: Cambridge University Press, 2009); George Gallup, "8 Out of 10 Favor 100 Million Fund for Heart Disease Study," *Washington Post*, June 26, 1948, 7.

3. T. D. Woolsey and I. M. Moriyama, "Statistical Studies of Heart Diseases: II. Important Factors in Heart Disease Mortality Trends," *Public Health Reports* 63, no. 39 (1948): 1247–1273; Mary Gover, "Statistical Studies of Heart Disease: IV. Mortality from Heart Disease (All Forms) Related to Geographic Section and Size of City," *Public Health Reports* 64, no. 14 (1949): 439–456; Mary Gover and Maryland Y. Pennell, "Statistical Studies of Heart Disease: VII. Mortality from Eight Specific Forms of Heart Disease among White Persons," *Public Health Reports* 65, no. 26 (1950): 819–838; I. M. Moriyama and T. D. Woolsey, "Statistical Studies of Heart Diseases: IX. Race and Sex Differences in the Trend of Mortality from the Major Cardiovascular-Renal Diseases," *Public Health Reports* 66, no. 12 (1951): 355–368. While these sources note that there was an apparent trend in cause-of-death attribution favoring coronary heart disease at the expense of stroke, there can be little doubt that CHD was genuinely increasing in prevalence as a cause of death.

4. Fye, *American Cardiology*, chap. 5; Theodore Van Dellen, "How to Keep Well," *Chicago Tribune*, April 9, 1948, 14; "Heart Disease Cost to Business Is Set at 2 Billion a Year," *Chicago Tribune*, January 2, 1949, SW14.

5. Oscar Ewing, "Wanted: Better Public Health," *Parade*, May 2, 1948, 5–7.

6. Louis I. Dublin to Leroy Lincoln, December 2, 1947 (quote); Dublin to Oscar Ewing, February 8, 1945; Dublin to William Shepard, March 2, 1948, all in folder National Health Assembly (Corres[pondence]) 1947–49, box 18, Louis I. Dublin Papers 1906–1968, MS C 316, Modern Manuscripts Collection, History of Medicine Division, US National Library of Medicine, Bethesda, MD; Editorial, "Mr. Ewing's Ten Year Health Program," *Journal of the American Medical Association* 138, no. 4 (1948): 297–298. On pre-1948 efforts at health reform, see Daniel M. Fox, *Power and Illness: The Failure and Future of American Health Policy* (Berkeley: University of California Press, 1993), chap. 2; Monte Poen, *Harry S. Truman versus the Medical Lobby: The Genesis of Medicare* (Columbia: University of Missouri Press, 1996); Jaap Kooijman, . . . *And the Pursuit of National Health: The Incremental Strategy toward National Health Insurance in the United States of America* (Atlanta, GA: Rodopi, 1999); Alan Derickson, *Health Security for All: Dreams of Universal Health Care in America* (Baltimore: Johns Hopkins University Press, 2005).

7. "Voluntary Health Agencies," 1944, folder 10, box 105, file PSF General, Truman Papers. On the NCI, see James Patterson, *The Dread Disease: Cancer and Modern American Culture* (Cambridge, MA: Harvard University Press, 1987); on the NFIP, see Angela Creager, "Mobilizing Biomedicine: Virus Research between Lay Health Organizations and the United States Federal Government, 1935–1955," in *Biomedicine in the 20th Century: Practices, Policies, and Politics*, ed. C. Hannaway (Amsterdam: IOS Press, 2008), 171–201; Daniel J. Wilson, "Basil O'Connor, the National Foundation for Infantile Paralysis and the Reorganization of Polio Research in the United States, 1935–41," *Journal of the History of Medicine and Allied Sciences* 70, no. 3 (2015): 394–424.

8. Fye, *American Cardiology*, chap. 2.

9. Harold Marvin to Paul Dudley White, September 30, 1942, folder 41, box 12; Marvin to White, August 10, 1943, folder 40, box 12, both in Paul Dudley White Papers, 1870s–1987, H MS c36, Harvard Medical Library, Francis A. Countway Library of Medicine, Boston, MA (hereafter, White Papers); Fye, *American Cardiology*, chap. 3.

10. Harold Marvin, "Conference with Dr. David Rutstein," April 14, 1943, folder 38, box 12, White Papers; Peter English, *Rheumatic Fever in America and Britain: A Biological, Epidemiological, and Medical History* (New Brunswick, NJ: Rutgers University Press, 1999).

11. Harold Marvin, "Conference with Dr. Haven Emerson," April 28, 1943, folder 38, box 3, and Marvin, "Conference with Dr. CEA Winslow," August 27, 1943, folder 40, box 12, both in White Papers.

12. Harold Marvin to Paul Dudley White, August 10, 1943, folder 40; Marvin, "Minutes of the Meeting of the Executive Committee," December 8, 1943, folder 42; Marvin, "Second Meeting of the Board of Directors, American Heart Association, Tuesday 8 February 1944," folder 44; and "Rheumatic Fever Conference, Hotel Lexington, January 26th and 27th, 1944, List of Participants," folder 44, all in box 12, White Papers.

13. Harold Marvin, "Memorandum relating to the Council on Rheumatic Fever," August 15, 1944, folder 47; "Meeting of the Executive Committee, American Heart Association, Wednesday November 29, 1944," folder 48; "Minutes of the Meeting of the American Council on Rheumatic Fever, Hotel Lexington, New York City, May 8, 1945," folder 49, all in box 12, White Papers.

14. David Rutstein, "Need for a Public Health Program in Rheumatic Fever and Rheumatic Heart Disease," *American Journal of Public Health* 36, no. 5 (1946): 461–467 (screening agency); Rutstein, "The Rheumatic Fever Community Program: Its Value in the Epidemiological Study of Rheumatic Fever: Summary of the Symposium," *American Journal of Public Health* 38, no. 8 (1948): 1082–1084 (careful integration); Rutstein with Homer F. Swift and Louis Speaker, "Approaches to the Rheumatic Fever Problem," n.d. [ca. 1946], folder 56, box 12, White Papers; Daniel M. Fox, "From TB to AIDS: Value Conflicts in Reporting Disease," *Hastings Center Report* 16, no. 6 (1986): 11–16.

15. W. D. King to Paul Dudley White, December 27, 1943, folder 42, box 12, White Papers; Howard A. Rusk, "Nation's Greatest Killer—Heart Disease—Challenged," *New York Times*, February 9, 1947, 4. The quote is from White, abstract of "Heart Disease: A World Problem," Hermann Biggs lecture of April 4, 1940, folder 42, box 12, White Papers. See also Paul Dudley White, "Climate, Mode of Life, and Heart Disease," *Annals of Internal Medicine* 12, no. 1 (1938): 6–12.

16. David Rutstein to Paul Dudley White, August 6, 1946, and Harold Marvin, Memorandum to Board of Directors, September 23, 1946, both in folder 56, box 12, White Papers.

17. Vannevar Bush, *Science, the Endless Frontier: A Report to the President* (Washington, DC: Government Printing Office, 1945); G. Pascal Zachary, *Endless Frontier: Vannevar Bush, Engineer of the American Century* (New York: Free Press, 1997), chap. 10.

18. Daniel J. Kevles, "The National Science Foundation and the Debate over Postwar Research Policy, 1942–1945: A Political Interpretation of Science—the Endless Frontier," *Isis* 68, no. 1 (1977): 5–26; Stephen Strickland, *The Story of the NIH Grants Programs* (Lanham, MD: University Press of America, 1989); Daniel Kleinman, "Layers of Interests, Layers of Influence: Business and the Genesis of the National Science Foundation," *Science, Technology and Human Values* 19, no. 3 (1994): 259–282.

19. "Minutes of Meeting of the Board of Directors, Barclay Hotel, New York City, October 18, 1945," folder 51, box 12; David Rutstein to Paul Dudley White, May 7, 1946, and attached statement by Duckett Jones before Senate Committee on Education and Labor concerning bill S.1606, April 26, 1946; "Statement Presented by Dr. David D. Rutstein . . . at the Hearings on H.R. 3922 before Subcommittee on Aid to the Physically Handicapped of the US House of Representatives, June 7, 1946," all in folder 55, box 12, White Papers.

20. David Rutstein, "Approaches to the Rheumatic Fever Problem," n.d. [ca. 1946], folder 56; "Minutes of the Executive Committee of the American Council on Rheumatic Fever of 8 April 1947," folder 57; "Minutes of the Meeting of the Executive Committee of the American Heart Association, May 4, 1947," folder 57, all in box 12, White Papers.

21. Fye, *American Cardiology*, chap. 3; "Minutes of the Meeting of the Board of Directors, American Heart Association of 8 June, 1947," folder 57, box 12, White Papers.

22. Fye, *American Cardiology*, chap. 3; Stephen Strickland, *Politics, Science, and Dread Disease: A Short History of United States Medical Research Policy* (Cambridge, MA: Harvard University Press, 1972); Strickland, *Story of the NIH Grants Programs*; Ronald Hamowy, *Government and Public Health in America* (Northampton, England: Edward Elgar, 2008); Hamilton Moses et al., "The Anatomy of Medical Research: US and International Comparisons," *Journal of the American Medical Association* 313, no. 2 (2015): 174–189.

23. See, for example, "Second Deficiency Appropriation Bill for 1948," Hearings before the Subcommittee of the Committee on Appropriations, US Senate, 80th Cong., 2nd sess., H.R. 6935, An Act Making Appropriations to Supply Deficiencies in Certain Appropriations for the Fiscal Year Ending June 30, 1948, and for Other Purposes, 137–142.

24. "National Heart Institute, 1950 Budget Estimates, Allowances, and Requirements," n.d. [ca. late 1949], spreadsheet, folder 72, box 3, White Papers. The NIH final budget figures are from "Appropriations History by Institute/Center (1938 to Present)," National Institutes of Health, http://officeofbudget.od.nih.gov/approp_hist.html. On White, see Oglesby Paul, *Take Heart: The Life and Prescription for Living of Paul Dudley White* (Cambridge, MA: Harvard University Press, 1986); J. Willis Hurst, "Paul Dudley White: The Father of American Cardiology," *Clinical Cardiology* 14, no. 7 (1991): 622–626; Clarence G. Lasby, *Eisenhower's Heart Attack: How Ike Beat Heart Disease and Held on to the Presidency* (Lawrence: University Press of Kansas, 1997).

25. See "Conference Structure," in "National Conference on Cardiovascular Diseases, January 18–20, 1950," 3–4, folder 67, box 3, White Papers.

26. A. Master, "Incidence of Acute Coronary Artery Occlusion: A Discussion of the Factors Responsible for Its Increase," *American Heart Journal* 33, no. 2 (1947): 135–145; Woolsey and Moriyama, "Statistical Studies of Heart Diseases: II," 1247–1273; Gover and Pennell, "Statistical Studies of Heart Disease: VII," 819–838; Moriyama and Woolsey, "Statistical Studies of Heart Diseases: IX," 355–368.

27. Menard M. Gertler, Stanley Marion Garn, and Paul Dudley White, "Diet, Serum Cholesterol and Coronary Artery Disease," *Circulation* 2, no. 5 (1950): 696–704. On changing assessments of dietary and serum cholesterol, see Todd Olszewski, "The Causal Conundrum: The Diet-Heart Debates and the Management of Uncertainty in American Medicine," *Journal of the History of Medicine and Allied Sciences* 70, no 2 (2014): 218–249. On theories of atherosclerosis and infarction, see David Jones, *Broken Hearts: The Tangled History of Cardiac Care* (Baltimore: Johns Hopkins University Press, 2013).

28. Louis I. Dublin with Herbert H. Marks, "The Influence of Weight on Certain Causes of Death," *Human Biology* 2, no. 2 (1930): 159–184; Emma Seifrit Weigley, "Average? Ideal? Desirable? A Brief Overview of Height-Weight Tables in the United States," *Journal of the American Dietetic Association* 84, no. 4 (1984): 417–423; Metropolitan Life Insurance Company, "Ideal Weights for Men," *Statistical Bulletin of the Metropolitan Life Insurance Company* 23 (1942): 6–8.

29. Harold M. Frost, "Hypertension and Longevity," *Boston Medical and Surgical Journal* 193, no. 6 (1925): 241–251; A. M. Master, H. H. Marks, and S. Dack, "Hypertension in People over Forty," *Journal of the American Medical Association* 121, no. 16 (1943): 1251–1256.

30. G. L. Duff and G. L. McMillan, "Pathogenesis of Atherosclerosis," Report III-a, n.d. [ca. late 1949]; R. L. Levy, "Diseases of the Coronary Arteries," Report III-d, n.d. [ca. late 1949]; F. E. Kendall, "The Biochemistry of Atherosclerosis," Report III-b, n.d. [ca. late 1949], all in folder 63, box 3, White Papers; Olszewski, "Causal Conundrum," 218–249; Irvine Page, "Hypertension," Report of

the Subcommittee on Hypertension (Section I, Committee on Technical Knowledge and Applications, Subcommittee 4), n.d. [ca. January 1950], folder 62, box 3, White Papers (mental rest, 4).

31. Roy Grinker, "Psychiatry and Psychosomatic Medicine," Report VI-a 14, folder 65, n.d. [ca. 1950]; Robert Malmo, "Psychology," Report VI-a 13, n.d. [ca. 1950], folder 65; Mandel Cohen to Paul Dudley White, January 16, 1950, folder 59; "Subcommittee on Neurocirculatory Asthenia (Anxiety Neurosis, Neurasthenia, Effort Syndrome) and Other Psychoneuroses," n.d. [ca. December 1949], folder 64, all in box 3, White Papers; Meyer Friedman et al., "Changes in the Serum Cholesterol and Blood Clotting Time in Men Subjected to Cyclic Variation of Occupational Stress," *Circulation* 17, no. 5 (1958): 852–861. On White's views concerning "nervous tension" in hypertensive heart disease, compare the third (1945, 432) and fourth (1951, 468) editions of his textbook *Heart Disease* (New York: Macmillan). On psychosomatic medicine, see Anne Harrington, *The Cure Within: A History of Mind-Body Medicine* (New York: Norton, 2008).

32. Alexander Langmuir, "Epidemiology," n.d. [ca. 1950], Report VI-a 18, folder 65; memorandum, John W. Ferree to Editorial Committee, National Conference on Cardiovascular Diseases, February 20, 1950, 22, folder 69, both in box 3, White Papers. On Langmuir, see Myron G. Schultz and William Schaffner, "Alexander Duncan Langmuir," *Emerging Infectious Diseases* 21, no. 9 (2015): 1635–1637, doi:10.3201/eid2109.141445.

33. W. A. Brumfield, "Final Report, Community Services, Case Finding and Epidemiology," January 19, 1950, folder 68, box 3, White Papers.

34. Hirschel Nisonger, "Preliminary Summary, Section on Community Services, Committee on Lay Education and Prevention," n.d. [ca. January 1950], folder 66; Irving Wright, Lyman Duff, and Forrest Kendall, "Suggestions from Section 1 for Sections 2 and 3 Consideration," January 19, 1950, 1, folder 60, both in box 3, White Papers.

35. "Proposed Heart Disease Program Meeting Minutes," August 3, 1947, folder 24, box 50, David D. Rutstein Papers, 1916–1989, H MS c315, Harvard Medical Library, Francis A. Countway Library of Medicine, Boston, MA (hereafter, Rutstein Papers); Gerald Oppenheimer, "Becoming the Framingham Study, 1947–1950," *American Journal of Public Health* 95, no. 4 (2005): 602–610.

36. "Proposed Study of the Epidemiology of Cardiovascular Disease," n.d. [ca. 1947], folder 241, box 50, Rutstein Papers; "Heart Shadows Measured for War on Disease," *Chicago Tribune*, April 26, 1947, 18; Bert Boone to E. R. Coffey, September 5, 1947, Boone to Gilcin Meadors, September 5, 1947, and L. C. Robbins to Meadors, September 5, 1947, all in temporal folders, Framingham Study Historical Papers, National Heart, Lung, and Blood Institute, Bethesda, MD (hereafter, Framingham Papers).

37. W. Palmer Dearing and Alexander E. Turner, "Chest Fluorography with Portable X-Ray Equipment on 35mm Film," *Public Health Reports* 55, no. 52 (1940): 2369–2377; Francis Weber, "Community-Wide Chest X-Ray Surveys: I. An Introduction to the Problem," *Public Health Reports* 62, no. 18 (1947): 652–658; Lester Breslow, "Multiphasic Screening Examinations—an Extension of the Mass Screening Technique," *American Journal of Public Health* 40, no. 3 (1950): 274–278.

38. Vlado Getting to David Rutstein, September 24, 1947, and Rutstein to Donald Armstrong, September 26, 1947, both in folder 24, box 50, Rutstein Papers. On the Framingham tuberculosis demonstration, see Ralph C. Matson, "The Framingham Health and Tuberculosis Demonstration: 1. Community Prevention, Control, and Treatment of Diseases, as Carried Out at Framingham, Massachusetts, USA," *Lancet* 203, no. 5259 (1924): 1243–1244; Diane Hamilton, "Research and Reform: Community Nursing and the Framingham Tuberculosis Project, 1914–1923," *Nursing Research* 41, no. 1 (1992): 8–13. Framingham can be viewed not as a research project that Rutstein

tried to derail with his activism, as Oppenheimer and PHS hindsight would have it, but as an interwar new public health–style activist heart disease intervention, which was reshaped into mere research under conservative political pressure in the early 1950s.

39. J. A. Crabtree to David Rutstein, September 30, 1947; Rutstein to Thomas Parran, October 10, 1947; "Heart Disease Epidemiology Study," including "Agreement on Administrative Arrangements for Fiscal Year 1948," [ca. 1947], all in folder 24, box 50, Rutstein Papers; Gilcin Meadors to Office of Surgeon General, July 20, 1948 (quote), temporal folder, Framingham Papers. Meadors was reported as leading the "Heart Disease Epidemiology" study and Lewis Robbins the "Cardiovascular Hygiene Demonstration" in December 1947 in Meadors, "Report of Activities for the Month of December 1947," January 8, 1948, folder 24, box 50, Rutstein Papers. See also Oppenheimer, "Becoming the Framingham Study," 602–610.

40. Lewis Robbins to Bert Boone, October 22, 1947 (quote), temporal folder, Framingham Papers; Boone to Vlado Getting, December 10, 1947, folder 23, box 50, Rutstein Papers; Felix Moore to C. J. van Slyke, August 26, 1949, temporal folder, Framingham Papers. It appears that in addition to diet and anxiety, which were eliminated from the study design during the period when Rutstein and Getting were nominally Meadors's managers, heredity and occupation were dropped in 1949 when the study passed formally to NIH control. The exclusion of easily recordable occupation data, at least, fits with the critique by some historians that Framingham's design was inimical to social medicine because it only examined variables accessible to individual fee-for-service clinical interventions. Suzanne G. Haynes et al., "The Relationship of Psychosocial Factors to Coronary Heart Disease in the Framingham Study: I. Methods and Risk Factors," *American Journal of Epidemiology* 107, no. 5 (1978): 362–383; Gerald Oppenheimer, "Profiling Risk: The Emergence of Coronary Heart Disease Epidemiology in the United States (1947–70)," *International Journal of Epidemiology* 35, no. 3 (2006): 720–730; Élodie Giroux, "The Framingham Study and the Constitution of a Restrictive Concept of Risk Factor," *Social History of Medicine* 26, no. 1 (2013): 94–112.

41. On the Massachusetts cancer program, see Fox, *Power and Illness*, 46; George Bigelow and Herbert L. Lombard, "Experience with the Program of Cancer Control in Massachusetts," *American Journal of Public Health* 18, no. 4 (1928): 413–420. See also "Massachusetts Health Department Press Release," June 10, 1948, folder 23, box 50, Rutstein Papers.

42. "Outline of the Proposed Work and the Plan of Attack of the Heart Control Program," [handmarked September 3, 1948]; Lewis Robbins to David Rutstein, September 16, 1948, both in folder 25, box 46; George F. Bowers, "Proposed Endorsement of Heart Demonstration Program by Newton Medical Club," October 8, 1948, folder 38, box 50, all in Rutstein Papers.

43. Pearl A. Thoreson, "Minutes of the Third Meeting of the Subcommittee on Nutrition," May 6, 1949, folder 31, box 50, Rutstein Papers.

44. Thoreson, "Minutes of the Third Meeting"; [Robbins?], "Newton Heart Demonstration Program: A Summary of Activities," November 8, 1950, folder 31, box 50, Rutstein Papers; Mary O'Brien, "Newton's 'Gluttons Anonymous' Share Reduction Problems," *Boston Globe*, April 2, 1950, A20.

45. Egon Kattwinkel et al., "A Public Health Heart Program: First Report," May 24, 1949, folder 31, box 50 (Alcoholics Anonymous); David Rutstein, "Heart Disease Programs: Clinical Basis and Organizational Aspects," n.d.; "Modified from a Manuscript Prepared for Publication in *Administrative Medicine*, edited by Haven Emerson, New York: Thomas Nelson and Sons, 1949," both in folder 15, box 73, all in Rutstein Papers. See the results of group weight loss in E. Kattwinkel, E. M. Morris, and L. C. Robbins, "Progress Report of the Newton Heart Demonstration

Program," *New England Journal of Medicine* 243, no. 3 (1950): 115. See also Council on Foods and Nutrition, "Some Nutritional Aspects of Sugar, Candy, and Sweetened Carbonated Beverages," *Journal of the American Medical Association* 120, no. 10 (1942): 763–765 (thanks to Cristin Kearns for this reference).

46. "General Staff Meeting Minutes," January 27, 1950, folder 20, box 2, NIH Directors files, Manuscript Collection 536, US National Library of Medicine, Bethesda, MD.

47. Vlado Getting and Herbert Lombard, "The Evaluation of Pilot Clinics, the Mass Screening or Health Protection Programs," June 1952, folder 37, box 68, Rutstein Papers.

48. David Rutstein, Charles R. Williamson, and Felix E. Moore, "Heart Disease Case Finding by Means of 70 Millimeter Photofluorographic Films," *Circulation* 4, no. 5 (1951): 641–651; David Rutstein and Ernest Craige, "Screening Tests in Mass Surveys and Their Use in Heart Disease Case Finding," *Circulation* 4 (November 1951): 659–665.

49. David Rutstein, "Approaches to the Rheumatic Fever Problem," n.d. [ca. 1946], folder 56, box 12; Howard Sprague, "Summary Statement, Committee 1, Section 1," n.d. [ca. January 1950], 3 (quote), folder 60, box 3, both in White Papers.

50. Report by Albert L. Chapman in "Meeting of the National Advisory Heart Council Agenda and Minutes," June 7–8, 1949, and report by Frederick Gillick in "Meeting of the National Advisory Heart Council Agenda and Minutes," June 1–3, 1950, both in cabinet C, Henry Blackburn Private Collection, University Archives, University of Minnesota, Twin Cities; "Association News," *American Journal of Public Health* 40 (1950): 1192; C. L. Mache Jr., "The Charleston Heart Demonstration Program: A Preliminary Report," *Journal of the South Carolina Medical Association* 49 (October 1953): 268–269.

51. [Albert L. Chapman], PHS Heart Disease Control Branch, Division of Chronic Disease, "Report of Heart Disease Control Activities for Fiscal Year 1950," folder 38, box 50, Rutstein Papers; Lester Breslow, "An Historical Review of Multiphasic Screening," *Preventive Medicine* 2, no. 2 (1973): 177–196.

52. Albert L. Chapman, "The Concept of Multiphasic Screening," *Public Health Reports* 64, no. 42 (1949): 1311–1314, quote 1314.

53. Lester Breslow, "Multiphasic Screening in California," *Journal of Chronic Diseases* 2, no. 4 (1955): 375–383, quote 382; Getting and Lombard, "Evaluation of Pilot Clinics."

54. Poen, *Harry S. Truman versus the Medical Lobby*, chaps. 6–7, quotes 148–149.

55. "Minutes of Meeting, Committee on Cardiovascular Disease Control," November 12, 1948, 4 (quote), folder 38, box 50, Rutstein Papers.

56. Rutstein to W. Palmer Dearing, August 23, 1950, folder 36, box 50, Rutstein Papers.

57. Memorandum, Paul Dudley White to National Advisory Heart Council, October 4, 1950, and associated untitled action plan; and brochure "Multiple Screening" (Washington, DC: Government Printing Office, [ca. 1951]), 83-171133, PHS pub. 7, all in folder 35, box 50, Rutstein Papers.

58. US Public Health Service, Bureau of State Services, *State Heart Disease Control Programs: Selected Information Included in the State Public Health Plans Submitted by State Health Departments for Fiscal Years 1954 and 1955*, PHS pub. 406 (Washington, DC: Government Printing Office, May 1954).

59. Republican National Committee, "Part 1: The 26th Pennsylvania Congressional Election," n.d. [ca. 1950]; and Republican National Committee, n.d. [ca. 1950], attached to Mike Gorman to Donald Dawson, n.d. [ca. March 1951], 1 (quote), both in folder 1, box 575, file OF 103, Truman Papers; "Voters' Verdict," *Washington Post*, November 9, 1950, 12.

60. Correspondence cross-reference sheet, "Lasker, Mrs. Albert D.," October 26, 1951, with summary and president's reply, folder 1949–53 (3/3), box 576, file OF 103, Truman Papers. See also Poen, *Harry S. Truman versus the Medical Lobby*, chaps. 6–7; Breslow, "Historical Review of Multiphasic Screening," 177–196.

CHAPTER 4: Fighting Heart Disease One Calorie at a Time
in Cold War Suburbia

1. See exchange between Senator Donnell and Emerson Foote, "National Heart Institute," Hearings on S.720 and S.2215, Subcommittee of the Committee on Labor and Public Welfare, US Senate, 80th Cong., 2nd sess., April 8, 1948, 128–130.

2. Barkev Sanders, "Local Health Departments: Growth or Illusion?," *Public Health Reports* 74, no. 1 (1959): 13–20; Berwyn Mattison, "Financing," *American Journal of Public Health* 47, no. 11 (1957): 20–21, quote 21.

3. Memorandum, Harry Truman to Donald S. Dawson, February 20, 1951, folder Health Needs of the Nation, box 577, file OF 103, Truman Papers, Truman Library, Independence, MO; Paul B. Magnuson, "The President's Commission on the Health Needs of the Nation," *Journal of the American Medical Association* 150, no. 15 (1952): 1509–1510; L. A. Alesen, "The Health Needs of the Nation," *California Medicine* 77, no. 5 (1952): 344–348; Editorial, "Health Needs of the Nation," *American Journal of Public Health* 43, no. 3 (1953): 335–337.

4. Editorial, "Health Needs of the Nation," 336.

5. Ellen Schrecker, *Many Are the Crimes: McCarthyism in America* (Princeton, NJ: Princeton University Press, 1999), chap. 10; Joel Isaac, "The Human Sciences in Cold War America," *History Journal* 50, no. 3 (2007): 725–746; Nancy Krieger, *Epidemiology and the People's Health: Theory and Context* (Oxford: Oxford University Press, 2011), chap. 5; Allan Brandt and Martha Gardner, "Antagonism and Accommodation: Interpreting the Relationship between Public Health and Medicine in the United States during the 20th Century," *American Journal of Public Health* 90, no. 5 (2000): 707–715. For more background on American social sciences in the Cold War, see Mark Solovey, *Shaky Foundations: The Politics–Patronage–Social Science Nexus in Cold War America* (New Brunswick, NJ: Rutgers University Press, 2013).

6. Alan Petersen and Deborah Lupton, *The New Public Health: Health and Self in the Age of Risk* (London: Sage, 1996).

7. J. E. Sabin, "Joseph Hersey Pratt's Cost Effective Class Method and Its Contemporary Application: Some Problems in Biopsychosocial Innovation," *Psychiatry* 53, no. 2 (1990): 169–184; Charles T. Ambrose, "Joseph Hersey Pratt (1872–1956): An Early Proponent of Cognitive-Behavioural Therapy in America," *Journal of Medical Biography* 22, no. 1 (2014): 33–44.

8. Ben Shephard, *A War of Nerves: Soldiers and Psychiatrists, 1914–1994* (London: Jonathan Cape, 2000); Saul Scheidlinger, "The Group Psychotherapy Movement at the Millennium: Some Historical Perspectives," *International Journal of Group Psychotherapy* 50 (2000): 315–339.

9. Benjamin Kotkov, "Technique and Explanatory Concepts of Short-Term Group Psychotherapy," *Journal of Psychology* 28, no. 2 (1949): 370–371, quote 375. Apart from the emphasis on repressed fears and sexual urges, the therapist is imagined as a substitute father, which is standard in psychoanalytic "transference."

10. Albert L. Chapman, "Weight Control: A Simplified Concept," *Public Health Reports* 66, no. 23 (1951): 725–731; Benjamin Kotkov, "Experiences in Group Psychotherapy with the Obese," *Psychosomatic Medicine* 15, no. 3 (1953): 243–251; Marjorie Grant and Joseph Rosenthal, "Group

Psychotherapy for Weight Control Delivery," *Massachusetts Health Journal* 31 (May 1950): 8–9; Arnold Kurlander, "Group Therapy in Reducing: Two-Year Follow-Up of the Boston Pilot Study," *Journal of the American Dietetic Association* 29 (1953): 337–339. On differences in modes of group psychotherapy, see Scheidlinger, "Group Psychotherapy Movement," 315–339.

11. "Appetites Anonymous Urged for Fat People," *Los Angeles Times*, May 5, 1950, 1; H. I. Harvey and W. D. Simmons, "Weight Reduction: A Study of the Group Method: Preliminary Report," *American Journal of the Medical Sciences* 225, no. 6 (1953): 623–625.

12. W. D. Simmons, "The Group Approach to Weight Reduction: I. A Review of the Project," *Journal of the American Dietetic Association* 30, no. 5 (1954): 437–441.

13. J. I. Goodman, E. D. Schwartz, and L. Frankel, "Group Therapy of Obese Diabetic Patients," *Diabetes* 2, no. 4 (1953): 280–284.

14. Kurlander, "Group Therapy in Reducing," 337–339; L. J. Bowser et al., "Methods of Reducing: Group Therapy vs. Individual Clinic Interview," *Journal of the American Dietetic Association* 29, no. 12 (1953): 1193–1196.

15. Joseph Aub, "Obesity Lecture Notes from 1940s," folder 31, box 17, Joseph Aub Papers, Manuscript Collection H MS c169, Harvard Medical Library, Francis A. Countway Library of Medicine, Boston, MA; Gary Taubes and Cristin Kearns Couzens, "Big Sugar's Sweet Little Lies," *Mother Jones*, November–December 2012, http://www.motherjones.com/environment/2012/10/sugar-industry-lies-campaign. Note that sugar can be blamed under the standard excess calories theory of obesity, not just under the less accepted (especially in the 1950s) theory that sugar has specific obesogenic hormonal effects. See Gary Taubes, "The Science of Obesity: What Do We Really Know about What Makes Us Fat?," *British Medical Journal* 346 (April 2013), doi:10.1136/bmj.f1050; Benjamin Rosenthal, Michael Jacobson, and Marcy Bohm, "Professors on the Take," *Progressive* 40, no. 11 (1976): 42–47.

16. M. J. Ford, "The Group Approach to Weight Control," *American Journal of Public Health* 43 (August 1953): 997–1000 (report on the June 1952 conference); Minna Gutsch, "The Weight Control Program in the Smaller Community: An Opportunity to Improve Everyday Food Habits," *American Journal of Public Health* 43 (December 1953): 1568–1571. Also see Albert L. Chapman, "An Experiment with Group Conferences for Weight Reduction," *Public Health Reports* 68, no. 4 (1953): 439–440, another experiment presumably discussed at the meeting.

17. US Public Health Service, Bureau of State Services, *State Heart Disease Control Programs: Selected Information Included in the State Public Health Plans Submitted by State Health Departments for Fiscal Years 1954 and 1955*, PHS pub. 406 (Washington, DC: Government Printing Office, May 1954).

18. Ford, "Group Approach to Weight Control," 997.

19. Louis I. Dublin, "Overweight, America's #1 Health Problem," typescript, April 30, 1952, quotes 1, 3, folder Overweight, America's #1 Health Problem, box 19, Louis I. Dublin Papers 1906–1968, MS C 316, Modern Manuscripts Collection, History of Medicine Division, US National Library of Medicine, Bethesda, MD; Dublin, "Overweight: America's No. 1 Health Problem," *Today's Health*, September 1952, 18–21; Donald B. Armstrong et al., "Obesity and Its Relation to Health and Disease," *Journal of the American Medical Association* 147, no. 11 (1951): 1007–1014.

20. Armstrong et al., "Obesity and Its Relation to Health and Disease," 1007–1014.

21. Louis I. Dublin and Herbert H. Marks, "Mortality among Insured Overweights in Recent Years," *Transactions of the Association of Life Insurance Medical Directors of America* 35 (1951): 235–263; Armstrong et al., "Obesity and Its Relation to Health and Disease," quote 1013.

22. Clifford Barborka, "Present Status of the Obesity Problem," *Journal of the American Med-*

ical Association 147, no. 11 (1951): 1015–1019, quote 1016; "Unneeded Fat Hangs Heavy on ¼ of U.S.," *Chicago Tribune*, December 5, 1951, 1.

23. Dublin and Marks, "Mortality among Insured Overweights," 235–263; Louis I. Dublin, "Benefits of Reducing," *American Journal of Public Health* 43, no. 8 (1953): 993–996; Dublin, "Fat People Who Lose Weight Live Longer," n.d. [1952], folder 33, box 77, David D. Rutstein Papers, 1916–1989, H MS c315, Harvard Medical Library, Francis A. Countway Library of Medicine, Boston, MA (hereafter, Rutstein Papers).

24. David Rutstein, "Discussion of Dr. Louis I. Dublin's Paper 'Fat People Who Lose Weight Live Longer,'" October 1952, folder 33, box 77, Rutstein Papers.

25. "The Greatest Problem in Preventive Medicine in the USA Is OBESITY," PHS pub. 6, GPO 83-171156, n.d. [ca.1951], unpaginated, folder 36, box 50, Rutstein Papers.

26. *Cheers for Chubby* (Metropolitan Life Insurance Company, Jerry Fairbanks Productions, 1951), posted by Averyl Hill, January 24, 2014, https://www.youtube.com/watch?v=140SJAYFMw0.

27. David Halberstam, *The Fifties* (New York: Villard 1993); Lizabeth Cohen, *A Consumers' Republic: The Politics of Mass Consumption in Postwar America* (New York: Knopf, 2003); Elaine Tyler May, *Homeward Bound: American Families in the Cold War Era*, rev. ed. (New York: Basic, 2008); Eva Moskowitz, *In Therapy We Trust: America's Obsession with Self-Fulfillment* (Baltimore: Johns Hopkins University, 2001); Alan Petigny, *The Permissive Society: America, 1941–1965* (New York: Cambridge University Press, 2009); Lisa McGirr, *Suburban Warriors: The Origins of the New American Right* (Princeton, NJ: Princeton University Press, 2015).

28. Helen Laville, "'If the Time Is Not Ripe, Then It Is Your Job to Ripen the Time!' The Transformation of the YWCA in the USA from Segregated Association to Interracial Organization, 1930–1965," *Women's History Review* 15, no. 3 (2006): 359–383.

29. Martha E. Gentry and Florence L. Swanson, "A Psychological Approach to Weight Control," *American Journal of Nursing* 52, no. 7 (1952): 849–850, quote 849.

30. Gentry and Swanson, "Psychological Approach to Weight Control," 849–850; Howard Wilson, "Weight in the YMCA Health Program," 1955, folder Wilson, Howard, box 27; "Minutes, Fourth Quarterly Meeting, 19/10/56," and attached appendix [1956]; John W. Ferree, "Current Work and Plans of the American Heart Association: Minutes, First Quarterly Meeting, 18/1/57," both in folder National YMCA Physical Education Committee Minutes, box 11, all in National YMCA Papers, University of Minnesota Archives, Minneapolis (documents courtesy of Jessica Parr); Jessica Parr, "We Lose Together: The Group Weight Control Movement in the United States, 1948 to 1970," PhD diss., University of New South Wales, 2018, chap. 3.

31. Parr, "We Lose Together," chap. 3.

32. Parr, "We Lose Together"; US Public Health Service, Bureau of State Services, *State Heart Disease Control Programs*, 19 (quote).

33. "TOPS, Born in Wisconsin, Depends on MD Guidance and Counsel," *Wisconsin Medical Journal* (January 1958): 79.

34. Parr, "We Lose Together," chap. 2. See also Samuel Wagonfeld and Howard M. Wolowitz, "Obesity and the Self-Help Group: A Look at TOPS," *American Journal of Psychiatry* 125, no. 2 (1968): 249–252; "TOPS Take[s] Off Pounds," *Life*, April 9, 1951, 137–140; Jack M'Curdy, "They Help Each Other," *Los Angeles Times*, September 6, 1959, CS1 (pig song).

35. Percy L. Smith, "Alcoholics Anonymous," *Psychiatric Quarterly* 15, no. 3 (1941): 554–562; Harry M. Tiebout, "Therapeutic Mechanisms of Alcoholics Anonymous," *American Journal of Psychiatry* 100, no. 4 (1944): 468–473; Robert Heath, "Group Therapy," *Psychosomatic Medicine* 8, no. 2 (1946): 118; L. Erwin Wexberg, "Outpatient Treatment of Alcoholics," *American Journal of*

Psychiatry 104, no. 9 (1948): 569–572; W. William, "The Society of Alcoholics Anonymous," *American Journal of Psychiatry* 105, no. 5 (1949): 370–375.

36. Jack Alexander, "Alcoholics Anonymous," *Saturday Evening Post*, March 1, 1941, 9–11, 89–92; William L. White, *Slaying the Dragon: The History of Addiction Treatment and Recovery in America* (Bloomington, IL: Lighthouse Institute, 1998); Mariana Valverde, *Diseases of the Will: Alcohol and the Dilemmas of Freedom* (Cambridge: Cambridge University Press, 1998).

37. Valverde, *Diseases of the Will*. Paul Ricoeur is among the scholars who have noted the congruence of psychoanalysis and Christian confession. See Ricoeur, *Freud and Philosophy*, trans. Denis Savage (New Haven, CT: Yale University Press 1970); Paul Rigby, "Paul Ricoeur, Freudianism, and Augustine's 'Confessions,'" *Journal of the American Academy of Religion* 53, no. 1 (1985): 93–114. Bill W.'s original Twelve Steps from chapter 5 of his 1938 manuscript, the basis of AA's early expansion and little changed since, can be found at http://silkworth.net/pages/originalmanuscript/chapter5.php (accessed August 2, 2018).

38. Antoinette Donnelly, "Fatties Anonymous: A New Way to Reduce," *Chicago Tribune*, October 12, 1950, C1; Donnelly, "First Week's Program and 10 Commandments of Fatties Anonymous," *Chicago Tribune*, October 13, 1950, B1; Wagonfeld and Wolowitz, "Obesity and the Self-Help Group," 249–252. On pastoral psychology and the gospel of self-fulfillment, see Petigny, *Permissive Society*; Moskowitz, *In Therapy We Trust*.

39. Antoinette Donnelly, "Success of Program in Fatties Anonymous Is Up to Individual," *Chicago Tribune*, October 14, 1950, B3 (shiftless, merry, tent-size, alibis); Donnelly, "Fat Persons' Irritation with Others Reflects Irritation with Selves," *Chicago Tribune*, October 18, 1950, B5 (know thyself); Donnelly, "Diet Plays Vital Role in Fatties Anonymous: Here Are First Menus," *Chicago Tribune*, October 16, 1950, D1 (inner conflicts); Parr, "We Lose Together," chap. 5.

40. *Beyond Our Wildest Dreams: A History of Overeaters Anonymous as Seen by a Cofounder* (Rio Rancho, NM: Overeaters Anonymous, 2005); Parr, "We Lose Together," chap. 5.

41. Donnelly, "Success of Program in Fatties Anonymous," B3 (rebirth); Nan Ickeringill, "Weight Watchers, Inc.: They Talk Their Way Out of Obesity," *New York Times*, March 20, 1967, 34.

42. Ickeringill, "Weight Watchers," 34; Louis Calta, "New Magazine Aims to Help the Overweight," *New York Times*, January 18, 1968, 36; "Jean Nidetch, 91, Is Dead: Founded Weight Watchers," *New York Times*, April 30, 2015, A1.

43. In 1960 diabetes was the eighth most common cause of death among American white women (seventh among nonwhite women) and accounted for about 10 percent of deaths among women attributed to heart disease and a much smaller proportion among men. US Department of Health, Education, and Welfare, *Vital Statistics of the United States, 1960*, vol. 2: *Mortality, Part A* (Washington, DC: Government Printing Office, 1963), https.//www.cdc.gov/nchs/data/vsus/VSUS_1960_2A.pdf, fig. 1-2.

44. Tavia Gordon, "Blood Pressure of Adults by Race and Area, United States, 1960–1962," *Vital and Health Statistics Data from the National Health Survey*, ser. 11, no. 5 (1964): 1–20; Caroline C. Garst, "Blood Glucose Levels in Adults: United States, 1960–1962," *Vital and Health Statistics Data from the National Health Survey*, ser. 11, no. 18 (1973): 1–25. Parr, "We Lose Together," chap. 4, finds evidence that TOPS included African American women in the later 1950s, mainly in segregated chapters. Evidence for male participation is scant before the late 1960s.

45. Fred Greenstein, *The Hidden-Hand Presidency: Eisenhower as Leader* (Baltimore: Johns Hopkins University Press, 1994).

46. "FDA's $648,000 Budget Cut," *FDC Reports*, May 30, 1953, W1–2; "FDA's Budget," *FDC Reports*, November 6, 1954, P3; "More FDA Inspections," *FDC Reports*, January 24, 1955, 1; Daniel

Carpenter, *Reputation and Power: Organizational Image and Pharmaceutical Regulation at the FDA* (Princeton, NJ: Princeton University Press, 2010), 167–169; Editorial, "The Federal Food and Drug Administration and the Public Health," *American Journal of Public Health* 45 (1955): 929–931; Glenn G. Slocum, "Pure Foods—Safe Drugs: The Food and Drug Administration's Role in Public Health," *American Journal of Public Health* 46, no. 8 (1956): 973–977.

47. Jack Haldeman, "The Changing Federal Role in Financing State and Local Health Services," *American Journal of Public Health* 45 (1955): 965–973.

48. "Are We Becoming Soft? Why the President Worries about Our Fitness," *Newsweek*, September 26, 1955, 35–36.

49. "Are We Becoming Soft?"; Hans Kraus and Ruth Prudden Hirschland, "Minimum Muscular Fitness Tests in School Children," *Research Quarterly for the American Association for Health, Physical Education and Recreation* 25, no. 2 (1954): 178–188, quote 178.

50. "Is American Youth Physically Fit?," *U.S. News and World Report*, August 2, 1957, 66–77 (fat and flabby); "Are We Becoming Soft?," 35–36; William Conklin, "Lack of Physical Fitness in U.S. Blasted by Government Official," *New York Times*, December 14, 1956, 48 (cushions); Donald P. Zingale, "'Ike' Revisited on Sport and National Fitness," *Research Quarterly for the American Association for Health, Physical Education and Recreation* 48, no. 1 (1977): 12–18.

51. "Are We Becoming Soft?," 35–36. That fitness was understood as the opposite of softness is clear from opponents of the youth fitness initiative too; see June Moser, "Our Children Are Not Softies," *Chicago Tribune*, February 3, 1957, F35. On the cultural aspects of bodily hardness, see Robert Corber, *Homosexuality in Cold War America: Resistance and the Crisis of Masculinity* (Durham, NC: Duke University Press, 1997); Robert L. Griswold, "The 'Flabby American,' the Body, and the Cold War," in *A Shared Experience: Men, Women, and the History of Gender*, ed. Laura McCall and Donald Yacovone (New York: New York University Press, 1998), 321–348; Kyle A. Cuordileone, "'Politics in an Age of Anxiety': Cold War Political Culture and the Crisis in American Masculinity, 1949–1960," *Journal of American History* 87, no. 2 (2000): 515–545; David K. Johnson, *The Lavender Scare: The Cold War Persecution of Gays and Lesbians in the Federal Government* (Chicago: University of Chicago Press, 2004); Jeffrey Montez De Oca, "'As Our Muscles Get Softer, Our Missile Race Becomes Harder': Cultural Citizenship and the 'Muscle Gap,'" *Journal of the History of Sociology* 18, no. 3 (2005): 145–172.

52. Frances Stonor Saunders, *Who Paid the Piper? The CIA and the Cultural Cold War* (London: Granta, 1999); Kenneth Osgood, *Total Cold War: Eisenhower's Secret Propaganda Battle at Home and Abroad* (Lawrence: University Press of Kansas, 2006). On biology and science generally in the Cold War, see Nicolas Rasmussen, *Gene Jockeys: Life Science and the Rise of Biotech Enterprise* (Baltimore: Johns Hopkins University Press), chap. 1. On sports, see Griswold, "The 'Flabby American,'" 321–348; De Oca, "As Our Muscles Get Softer," 145–172.

53. "If Russia Wins Olympic Games," *U.S. News and World Report*, February 10, 1956, 35–39, quotes 36, folder 156-A-6, box 703, file White House Central Official File 1953–61, Eisenhower Presidential Library, Abilene, KS (hereafter, Eisenhower Papers).

54. "Are We Becoming Soft?," 35–36; "President Eisenhower and 32 Sports Leaders Seek Means to Promote Physical Fitness," *Amateur Athlete*, August 1955, 4; "Conference on the Fitness of American Youth, 27–28 September 1955," unpaginated conference program, folder 156-A-6, box 703, file White House Central Official File 1953–61, box 703, Eisenhower Papers; Bill Armstrong, "President's Council on American Youth," *Amateur Athlete*, July 1956, 6; "Ike to Appoint Council to Boost Fitness of Youth," *Chicago Tribune*, June 20, 1956, 3 (overriding); Matthew T. Bowers and Thomas M. Hunt, "The President's Council on Physical Fitness and the Systematisa-

tion of Children's Play in America," *International Journal of the History of Sport* 28, no. 11 (2011): 1496–1511.

55. "President's Group Urges Play Streets," *Washington Post and Times Herald*, November 30, 1956, B1; Homer Bigart, "Youth Fitness Aid Favored by Nixon," *New York Times*, September 10, 1957, 66; Harry Gabbett, "Youth Fitness via Adults Urged," *Washington Post*, July 31, 1957, A22; Shane McCarthy, "Fitness Week," *Washington Post*, June 2, 1958, A12; "Total Fitness Stressed for Youth Week," *Washington Post*, May 3, 1959, B1.

56. Marcia Winn, "Easy Way to More Muscle: Some Schools Developing Fitness," *Chicago Tribune*, November 5, 1957, A1; "Americans 'Overfed, Unfit,'" *Washington Post*, June 6, 1957, D3 (husbands moving).

57. Patricia A. Eisenman and C. Robert Barnett, "Physical Fitness in the 1950s and 1970s: Why Did One Fail and the Other Boom?," *Quest* 31 (1979): 114–117; Bowers and Hunt, "President's Council on Physical Fitness," 1496–1511; Zingale, "'Ike' Revisited on Sport and National Fitness," 12–18.

CHAPTER 5: The New Epidemiology and Its Impact

1. CBS Television Network, "CBS Reports: The Fat American Script," January 18, 1962, 1, 6, 2, 16, 31 (quotes), folder 1, box 4, Paul Dudley White Papers, 1870s–1987, H MS c36, Harvard Medical Library, Francis A. Countway Library of Medicine, Boston, MA.

2. Ancel Keys, "Overweight and Reducing," n.d. [ca. 1977], 1–2, 6–7 (quotes), cabinet H, file Drafts, Overweight and Reducing, Henry Blackburn Private Collection, University Archives, University of Minnesota, Twin Cities (hereafter, Blackburn Collection).

3. Halbert L. Dunn, *Vital Statistics of the United States, 1950* (Washington, DC: Government Printing Office, 1954), https://www.cdc.gov/nchs/data/vsus/vsus_1950_1.pdf. Tables 8.42 and 8.43 show that on an age-adjusted basis, for white males deaths attributed to "arteriosclerotic heart disease" alone accounted for about 30 percent of all deaths, while for the entire population (all races and sexes) deaths from "arteriosclerotic heart disease" combined with "general arteriosclerosis" and "hypertension with heart disease" accounted for a third of all deaths in 1950. T. D. Woolsey and I. M. Moriyama, "Statistical Studies of Heart Diseases: II. Important Factors in Heart Disease Mortality Trends," *Public Health Reports* 63, no. 39 (1948): 1247–1273; Mary Gover and Maryland Y. Pennell, "Statistical Studies of Heart Disease: VII. Mortality from Eight Specific Forms of Heart Disease among White Persons," *Public Health Reports* 65, no. 26 (1950): 819–838; I. M. Moriyama and T. D. Woolsey, "Statistical Studies of Heart Disease: IX. Race and Sex Differences in the Trend of Mortality from the Major Cardiovascular-Renal Diseases," *Public Health Reports* 66, no. 12 (1951): 355–368. Also see Tavia Gordon and Thomas Thom, "The Recent Decrease in CHD Mortality," *Preventive Medicine* 4, no. 2 (1975): 115–125, fig. 1.

4. Jeanne Truett, Jerome Cornfield, and William Kannel, "A Multivariate Analysis of the Risk of Coronary Heart Disease in Framingham," *Journal of Chronic Diseases* 20, no. 7 (1967): 511–524; Élodie Giroux, "The Framingham Study and the Constitution of a Restrictive Concept of Risk Factor," *Social History of Medicine* 26, no. 1 (2013): 94–112.

5. Henry Blackburn and David Jacobs Jr., "Commentary: Origins and Evolution of Body Mass Index (BMI): Continuing Saga," *International Journal of Epidemiology* 43, no. 3 (2014): 665–669, quote 667.

6. Ancel Keys et al., "Coronary Heart Disease among Minnesota Business and Professional Men Followed Fifteen Years," *Circulation* 28, no. 3 (1963): 381–395, quote 386.

7. Ancel Keys et al., *Experimental Starvation in Man* (Arlington, VA: Air Force Office of Scientific Research, 1945); Henry Blackburn, "Introduction to Ancel Keys Lecture: Ancel Keys, Pioneer," *Circulation* 84, no. 3 (1991): 1402–1404; Todd Tucker, *The Great Starvation Experiment: The Heroic Men Who Starved So That Millions Could Live* (New York: Simon and Schuster, 2006). Keys found that semi-starvation led to impaired heart function and a greater proportional weight loss from vitally important tissues than from fat tissue. (This study on starvation could imply that weight loss, as in dieting, might be harmful to the heart, but logically says nothing about the effects of excess food consumption.) He also conducted work on the effects of hormones on metabolism and some mostly unpublished studies that led him to design a health-maintaining lightweight diet for soldiers, which was realized as the "K ration." I found no published work by Keys prior to the late 1940s specifically linking the intake of particular fats to indicators of health status.

8. Ancel Keys, "Obesity and Degenerative Heart Disease," *American Journal of Public Health* 44 (July 1954): 864–871. Blackburn and Jacobs recalled that the insurance studies "irritated" Keys throughout his entire career, although I found published evidence of this only after the war. Another argument Keys often made against the insurance statistics is that only overweight people who knew they were at risk of early death would buy insurance despite the higher rate penalty. While adverse selection of some kind is plausible, it does not apply to the period before moderate overweight attracted higher premiums, when the industry first characterized the impairment. Moreover Keys offered no explanation of how overweight people could know that they were particularly likely to die from cardiovascular disease but not other causes (which would be required to account for the statistics of analysts like Dublin). Blackburn and Jacobs, "Commentary: Origins and Evolution of Body Mass Index," 665–669.

9. Cristin E. Kearns, Laura A. Schmidt, and Stanton A. Glantz, "Sugar Industry and Coronary Heart Disease Research: A Historical Analysis of Internal Industry Documents," *JAMA Internal Medicine* 176, no. 11 (2016): 1680–1685. Gary Taubes and Cristin Kearns Couzens, "Big Sugar's Sweet Little Lies," *Mother Jones*, November–December 2012, http://www.motherjones.com/environment/2012/10/sugar-industry-lies-campaign; and Taubes, *The Case against Sugar* (New York: Knopf, 2016), 129, report that both Fred Stare and Ancel Keys received sugar funding during the "war years." In 1945 both Stare and Keys enjoyed large grants from the Sugar Research Foundation ($25,000 and $30,000, respectively). See *Some Facts about the Sugar Research Foundation Inc. and Its Prize Awards Program* (New York: Sugar Research Foundation, 1945) (thanks to Cristin Kearns for this source). On the tobacco industry, see Robert Hockett to Edwin B. Wilson, April 7, 1958, and Edwin Bidwell Wilson to Robert Hockett, February 20, 1958? (sketchy), *Tobacco Industry Documents*, https://industrydocuments.library.ucsf.edu/tobacco/docs/xyjg0216 and https://industrydocuments.library.ucsf.edu/tobacco/docs/jyjg0216. See also Allan Brandt, *The Cigarette Century: The Rise, Fall, and Deadly Persistence of the Product That Defined America* (New York: Basic Books, 2007), chaps. 5–6; Robert Proctor, *Golden Holocaust: Origins of the Cigarette Catastrophe and the Case for Abolition* (Berkeley: University of California Press, 2011), chap. 16.

10. Ancel Keys, "Prediction and Possible Prevention of Coronary Disease," *American Journal of Public Health* 43 (1953): 1399–1407; Ancel Keys and Francisco Grande, "Role of Dietary Fat in Human Nutrition: III. Diet and the Epidemiology of Coronary Heart Disease," *American Journal of Public Health* 47 (1957): 1520–1530.

11. John Yudkin, "Diet and Coronary Thrombosis: Hypothesis and Fact," *Lancet* 270, no. 6987 (1957): 155–162; Taubes, *Case against Sugar*; David M. Johns and Gerald M. Oppenheimer, "Was There Ever Really a 'Sugar Conspiracy'?," *Science* 359, no. 6377 (2018): 747–750.

12. J. M. Chapman et al., "IV. The Clinical Status of a Population Group in Los Angeles under Observation for Two to Three Years," *American Journal of Public Health* 47, no. 4 (1957): 33–42; L. S. Goerke, John M. Chapman, and Edward Phillips, "Diseases of the Heart in a Working Population: A Study of Morbidity and Mortality in Relation to Cardiac Status and Nature of Job," *California Medicine* 87, no. 6 (1957): 398–402; Lester Breslow, *A Life in Public Health: An Insider's Retrospective* (New York: Springer, 2005), chap. 4.

13. Joseph T. Doyle et al., "A Prospective Study of Degenerative Cardiovascular Disease in Albany: Report of Three Years' Experience: 1. Ischemic Heart Disease," *American Journal of Public Health* 47, no. 4 (1957): 25–32; Joseph T. Doyle, "Early Diagnosis of Ischemic Heart Disease," *New England Journal of Medicine* 261, no. 22 (1959): 1096–1101; J. Stamler et al., "Prevalence and Incidence of Coronary Heart Disease in Strata of the Labor Force of a Chicago Industrial Corporation," *Journal of Chronic Diseases* 11, no. 3 (1960): 405–420.

14. Thomas R. Dawber, Felix E. Moore, and George V. Mann, "II. Coronary Heart Disease in the Framingham Study," *American Journal of Public Health* 47 (1957): 4–24. On the changing norms of blood pressure in the 1950s and especially the 1960s, see Jeremy Greene, *Prescribing by Numbers: Drugs and the Definition of Disease* (Baltimore: Johns Hopkins University Press, 2006).

15. Dawber, Moore, and Mann, "II. Coronary Heart Disease in the Framingham Study," 4–24, quote 15.

16. Dawber, Moore, and Mann, "II. Coronary Heart Disease in the Framingham Study," 18–19; Ancel Keys, "The Diet and the Development of Coronary Heart Disease," *Journal of Chronic Diseases* 4, no. 4 (1956): 364–380.

17. John J. Hutchinson, "Clinical Implications of an Extensive Actuarial Study of Build and Blood Pressure," *Annals of Internal Medicine* 54, no. 1 (1961): 90–96; Hutchinson, "Highlights of the New Build and Blood Pressure Study," *Transactions of the Association of Life Insurance Medical Directors of America* 43 (1959): 34–42, quote 36.

18. William B. Kannel et al., "Relation of Body Weight to Development of Coronary Heart Disease: The Framingham Study," *Circulation* 35 (1967): 734–744. Also see A. Kagan et al., "The Framingham Study: Prospective Study of Coronary Heart Disease," *Federation Proceedings* 21 (1962): 52–57.

19. M. Higgins et al., "III. Hazards of Obesity: The Framingham Experience," *Acta Medica Scandinavica*, suppl., 723 (1988): 23–36.

20. CBS Television Network, "CBS Reports: The Fat American Script."

21. Nicolas Rasmussen, *On Speed: The Many Lives of Amphetamine* (New York: New York University Press, 2008).

22. "The Liver of an Overweight Patient" (Smith, Kline and French advertisement) *California Medicine* 74, no. 6 (1951): n.p.; "One Disease That Doesn't Hurt" (Smith, Kline and French advertisement), *Journal of the American Medical Association* 151, no. 1 (1953): 41.

23. "When Temptation Makes a Fifth at Bridge" (Desoxyn advertisement), *Journal of the American Medical Association* 151, no. 16 (1953): 53; "Establishing Desired Eating Patterns" (Obedrin advertisement), *California Medicine* 83, no. 7 (1955): 22.

24. Desoxyn Gradumet advertisement in *Journal of the American Medical Association* 174, no. 3 (1960): 272–273; "Stick-to-It-Iveness Is Fine . . ." (Efroxine advertisement), *California and Western Medicine* 72, no. 6 (1950): 25; Roy Gibbons, "Tip to Fat Men: It Takes Courage to Shed Weight," *Chicago Tribune*, June 14, 1951, 1; Clifford Barborka, "Present Status of the Obesity Problem," *Journal of the American Medical Association* 147, no. 11 (1951): 1015–1019, quotes 1018 (courage), 105 (quick).

25. "Prescription: AmPlus Now" (AmPlus advertisement), *California Medicine* 82, no. 5 (1955): n.p.; "Predictable Weight Loss" (Biphetamine and Ionamin advertisement), *Journal of the American Medical Association* 174, no. 2 (1960): 35.

26. "I Know You're Right Doctor" (Efroxine advertisement), *Journal of the American Medical Association* 146, no. 5 (1951): 55; "Predictable Weight Loss," 135.

27. Memorandum, FDA inspector Dominic Ziccardi to Chief, New York District, May 8, 1958, re Reducing Drugs, 573–576, in US Senate, "The Diet Pill Industry," Hearings before the Subcommittee on Antitrust and Monopoly of the Committee on the Judiciary, US Senate, 19th Cong., 2nd sess., January 23, 24, 26, 30, 31 and February 2, 1968 (Washington, DC: Government Printing Office, 1968) (hereafter, "Diet Pill Industry").

28. "Specific Medication for the Disease of Obesity," Lanpar brochure, n.d., in "Diet Pill Industry," 466.

29. Hearings of Subcommittee on Health, Senate Committee on Labor and Public Welfare, Hearings on S.2628, 88th Cong., 2nd sess., March 12, 1964, 23–24; "Diet Pill Industry," 75, 91; George Burditt to Dorothy Goodwin, July 8, 1967, in "Diet Pill Industry," 467; Nicolas Rasmussen, "America's First Amphetamine Epidemic, 1929–1971: A Quantitative and Qualitative Retrospective with Implications for the Present," *American Journal of Public Health* 98, no. 6 (2008): 974–985; Pieter A. Cohen, Alberto Goday, and John P. Swann, "The Return of Rainbow Diet Pills," *American Journal of Public Health* 102, no. 9 (2012): 1676–1686.

30. L. B. Janis, "The Value of Amphetamine Compounds in the Medical Management of Obesity," *Ohio State Medical Journal* 51, no. 11 (1955): 1101–1102. It is not extravagant to estimate the number of Americans annually receiving amphetamines from fat doctors in the early 1960s as more than a million, if one allows that on average each of the 5,000 practitioners treated 200 different patients in a year. After all, the busier ones saw more than double that many patients in a week.

31. Israel Bram, "Psychic Factors in Obesity Observations in over 1,000 Cases," *Archives of Pediatrics* 67 (1950): 543–552, quote 545–546.

32. "Wyeth's Ansolysen," *FDC Reports*, September 1954, white-12.

33. R. J. Vakil, "A Clinical Trial of *Rauwolfia serpentina* in Essential Hypertension," *British Heart Journal* 11, no. 4 (1949): 350–355; N. K. Chakravarty and M. N. Chaudhuri, "*Rauwolfia serpentina* in Essential Hypertension," *Indian Medical Gazette* 86, no. 8 (1951): 348–354; R. W. Wilkins and W. E. Judson, "The Use of *Rauwolfia serpentina* in Hypertensive Patients," *New England Journal of Medicine* 248, no. 2 (1953): 48–53; J. Tripod, H. J. Bein, and R. Meier, "Characterization of Central Effects of Serpasil (Reserpin[e], a New Alkaloid of *Rauwolfia serpentina B.*) and of Their Antagonistic Reactions," *Archives Internationales de Pharmacodynamie et de Therapie* 96, nos. 3–4 (1954): 406–425; "Ciba's Serpasil," *FDC Reports*, March 1955, 11; "Tranquility Drug Market," *FDC Reports*, December 1955, 10–11; two-page advertisement for Ciba's Serpasil, *New England Journal of Medicine* 258, no. 1 (1958): n.p.; "For Total Management of Your Hypertensive Patients" (Raudixin [Squibb] advertisement), *New England Journal of Medicine* 258, no. 2 (1958): xv. Also see Judith P. Swazey, *Chlorpromazine in Psychiatry: A Study of Therapeutic Innovation* (Cambridge, MA: MIT Press, 1974); David Healy, *The Creation of Psychopharmacology* (Cambridge, MA: Harvard University Press, 2009), chap. 3.

34. The NAHC was concerned about hypertension, feeling that not enough researchers were studying it, but the council funded far more fat metabolism research. See "Meeting of the National Advisory Heart Council: Agenda and Minutes, 12–14 February 1953," 2–3, cabinet C, file Meeting Minutes February 12–14, 1953, Blackburn Collection.

35. "Hypertension Drug Evaluation," *FDC Reports*, November 26, 1956, 16; "Heart Drug Evaluation," *FDC Reports*, January 14, 1957, 15.

36. "Remarks Made by Leonard Scheele," February 28, 1958, 5; "Minutes of Meeting, February 27–28–March 1," 3, 12, both in "Meeting of the National Advisory Heart Council: Agenda and Minutes, 27 February–1 March 1958," cabinet C, file Meeting Minutes and Agenda (Alumni) February 27–March 1, 1958, Blackburn Collection.

37. Jeremy Greene, "Releasing the Flood Waters: Diuril and the Reshaping of Hypertension," *Bulletin of the History of Medicine* 79, no. 4 (2005): 749–794; "Diuril Competitive Race," *FDC Reports*, November 17, 1958, 21.

38. Ancel Keys and Margaret Keys, *Eat Well and Stay Well* (New York: Doubleday, 1959).

39. Frank P. Palopoli, "Basic Research Leading to MER-29," *Progress in Cardiovascular Diseases* 2, no. 6 (1960): 489–491; Ralph Adam Fine, *The Great Drug Deception: The Shocking Story of MER/29 and the Folks Who Gave You Thalidomide* (New York: Stein and Day, 1972), chaps. 4–5; William Hollander, Aram V. Chobanian, and Robert W. Wilkins, "The Effects of Triparanol (MER-29) in Subjects with and without Coronary Artery Disease," *Journal of the American Medical Association* 174, no. 1 (1960): 5–12; Nicolas Rasmussen, "The Drug Industry and Clinical Research in Interwar America: Three Types of Physician Collaborator," *Bulletin of the History of Medicine* 79, no. 1 (2005): 50–80.

40. Fine, *Great Drug Deception*, 66; "Rich-Merrell's MER-29," *FDC Reports*, October 30, 1961, 23.

41. "No Common Cold Vaccine," *FDC Reports*, September 28, 1959, 21; "Merrell's Anticholesterol Drug, MER-29, Is Coming in Big," *FDC Reports*, October 10, 1960, 23–24; "Richardson-Merrell's Foreign Sales Up $6.9 Mil.," *FDC Reports*, September 25, 1961, 8–10.

42. Fine, *Great Drug Deception*, chaps. 4–5.

43. Arthur A. Daemmrich, *Pharmacopolitics: Drug Regulation in the United States and Germany* (Chapel Hill: University of North Carolina Press, 2004).

44. Todd M. Olszewski, "The Causal Conundrum: The Diet-Heart Debates and the Management of Uncertainty in American Medicine," *Journal of the History of Medicine and Allied Sciences* 70, no. 2 (2014): 218–249.

45. Marion Nestle, *Food Politics: How the Food Industry Influences Nutrition and Health* (Berkeley: University of California Press, 2013), chap. 1.

46. Irvine H. Page et al., "Atherosclerosis and the Fat Content of the Diet," *Circulation* 16, no. 2 (1957): 163–178.

47. Herbert Pollack, "Editorial: Dietary Fats and Their Relationship to Atherosclerosis," *Circulation* 16, no. 2 (1957): 161–162.

48. S. M. Grundy et al., "Rationale of the Diet-Heart Statement of the American Heart Association," *Circulation* 65, no. 4 (1982): 839–854.

49. Ancel Keys and Seven Countries Investigators, "Coronary Heart Disease in Seven Countries: The Study Program and Objectives," *Circulation*, suppl., 41, no. S1 (1970): 1–8.

50. Irvine Page, "Editorial: The National Diet-Heart Study," *Circulation* 29, no. 1 (1964): 4–5; B. M. Baker et al., "The National Diet-Heart Study: An Initial Report," *Journal of the American Medical Association* 185, no. 2 (1963): 105–106; "The National Diet-Heart Study: Final Report," *Circulation*, suppl., 37, no. S3 (1969): 428. See also Harry Marks, *The Progress of Experiment: Science and Therapeutic Reform in the United States, 1900–1990* (Cambridge: Cambridge University Press, 2000), 181–196.

51. Ancel Keys and Seven Countries Investigators, "Coronary Heart Disease in Seven Coun-

tries: Summary," *Circulation*, suppl., 41, no. S1 (1970): 186–195; Keys et al., "Coronary Heart Disease in Seven Countries: The Diet," *Circulation*, suppl., 41, no. S1 (1970): 162–183; Keys et al., "Some Problems," *Circulation*, suppl., 41, no. S1 (1970): 184–185; H. L. Taylor et al., "Coronary Heart Disease in Seven Countries: IV. Five-Year Follow-Up of Employees of Selected U.S. Railroad Companies," *Circulation*, suppl., 41, no. S1 (1970): 20–39.

52. Keys et al., "Coronary Heart Disease in Seven Countries: Summary"; Keys et al., "Coronary Heart Disease in Seven Countries: The Diet"; Taylor et al., "Coronary Heart Disease in Seven Countries."

53. Louis I. Dublin, "Benefits of Reducing," *American Journal of Public Health* 43 (1953): 993–996.

CHAPTER 6: The Disappearance of Obesity as a Public Health Problem

1. Monte Poen, *Harry S. Truman versus the Medical Lobby: The Genesis of Medicare* (Columbia: University of Missouri Press, 1996); Allan Brandt, *The Cigarette Century: The Rise, Fall, and Deadly Persistence of the Product That Defined America* (New York: Basic Books, 2007); Robert N. Proctor, *Golden Holocaust: Origins of the Cigarette Catastrophe and the Case for Abolition* (Berkeley: University of California Press, 2011); "History of the Surgeon General's Reports on Smoking and Health," Centers for Disease Control and Prevention, last modified July 2009, https://www.cdc.gov/tobacco/data_statistics/sgr/history/index.htm.

2. I am thinking of the work of scholars Becker, Goffman, and Zola, despite the great differences among them. Howard S. Becker, *Outsiders: Studies in the Sociology of Deviance* (New York: Free Press, 1963); Erving Goffman, *Stigma: Notes on the Management of Spoiled Identity* (New York: Simon and Schuster, 1963); Irving Zola, "Medicine as an Institution of Social Control," *Sociological Review* 20, no. 4 (1972): 487–504.

3. Zola, "Medicine as an Institution of Social Control," 487–504; Peter Conrad, "Types of Medical Social Control," *Sociology of Health and Illness* 1, no. 1 (1979): 1–11.

4. Editorial, "The U.S. National Health Survey," *American Journal of Public Health* 48, no. 7 (1958): 923.

5. F. E. Linder, "National Health Survey: Established in 1956, It Is Measuring Levels, Trends, and Social Consequences of Various Illnesses," *Science* 127, no. 3309 (1958): 1275–1280.

6. Tavia Gordon, "Blood Pressure of Adults by Age and Sex, United States, 1960–1962," *Vital and Health Statistics Data from the National Health Survey*, ser. 11, no. 4 (1964): 1–40 (table F); Gordon, "Blood Pressure of Adults by Race and Area, United States, 1960–1962," *Vital and Health Statistics Data from the National Health Survey*, ser. 11, no. 5 (1964): 1–30 (table 3); Thomas R. Dawber, Felix E. Moore, and George V. Mann, "II. Coronary Heart Disease in the Framingham Study," *American Journal of Public Health* 47 (1957): 4–24, table 7.

7. Felix E. Moore and Tavia Gordon, "Serum Cholesterol Levels of Adults, United States, 1960–1962," *Vital and Health Statistics Data from the National Health Survey*, ser. 11, no. 22 (1967): 1–23 (table B); Dawber, Moore, and Mann, "II. Coronary Heart Disease in the Framingham Study," 4–24.

8. Jean Roberts, *Weight by Height and Age of Adults, United States, 1960–1962*, ser. 11, pub. 14 (Washington, DC: Government Printing Office, 1966); Society of Actuaries, *Build and Blood Pressure Study*, vol. 1 (Schaumburg, IL: Society of Actuaries, 1959).

9. "Unneeded Fat Hangs Heavy on ¼ of U.S.," *Chicago Tribune*, December 5, 1951, 1; Donald B. Armstrong et al., "Obesity and Its Relation to Health and Disease," *Journal of the American*

Medical Association 147, no. 11 (1951): 1007–1014. In the Armstrong article, 20 percent of the adult population were estimated to be overweight, defined as 10–19 percent above ideal weight for height, and an additional 5 percent were "pathologically obese" at 20 percent or more. Based on Roberts, *Weight by Height and Age of Adults*, table 5, if one takes the mean weight for eighteen- to twenty-four-year-olds at the median male height of sixty-eight inches as the ideal weight, in line with later PHS analyses, then the third quartile of men thirty-five to forty-four is delineated by almost exactly 120 percent of that weight. See, for example, S. Abraham et al., "Obese and Overweight Adults in the United States," *Vital and Health Statistics Data from the National Health Survey*, ser. 11, no. 230 (1983): 1–98.

10. Abraham et al., "Obese and Overweight Adults," 1–98. This study defined "ideal weight" differently than actuarial best weight, instead using median weight for height in the twenty to twenty-nine age group as the standard ideal weight for all age groups; overweight was now defined as the eighty-fifth percentile of weight for height for people in their twenties. Given that even Americans in their twenties were overweight by actuarial standards, this measure introduced a further narrowing in comparison to prior insurance studies and thus further minimized the apparent prevalence of overweight in the United States circa 1970 compared with 1950, although the insurance estimates of prevalence were admittedly not based on probability samples.

11. Abraham et al., "Obese and Overweight Adults," 4–5.

12. Abraham et al., "Obese and Overweight Adults," 1. See table 7 and compare table 1 from 1966.

13. Ancel Keys, the Committee on Nutritional Anthropometry, Food and Nutrition Board, and National Research Council, "Recommendations concerning Body Measurements for the Characterization of Nutritional Status," *Human Biology* 28, no. 2 (1956): 111–112; Ancel Keys et al., "Coronary Heart Disease among Minnesota Business and Professional Men Followed Fifteen Years," *Circulation* 28, no. 3 (1963): 381–395.

14. Josef Brozek, "Changes in Specific Gravity and Body Fat of Young Men under Conditions of Experimental Semi-starvation," *Federation Proceedings* 5, no. 1 (1946): 13; Henry Blackburn and David Jacobs Jr. "Commentary: Origins and Evolution of Body Mass Index (BMI): Continuing Saga," *International Journal of Epidemiology* 43, no. 3 (2014): 665–669; Keys et al., "Recommendations concerning Body Measurements," 111–112; Ancel Keys and Josef Brozek, "Body Fat in Adult Man," *Physiological Reviews* 33, no. 3 (1953): 245–325.

15. Herbert H. Marks, "Body Weight: Facts from Life Insurance Records," *Human Biology* 28, no. 2 (1956): 217–231.

16. Arnold B. Kurlander, Sidney Abraham, and J. Wallace Rion, "Obesity and Disease," *Human Biology* 28, no. 2 (1956): 203–216.

17. Ancel Keys and Seven Countries Investigators, "Coronary Heart Disease in Seven Countries: Summary," *Circulation*, suppl., 41, no. S1 (1970): 186–195.

18. Ancel Keys et al., "Coronary Heart Disease: Overweight and Obesity as Risk Factors," *Annals of Internal Medicine* 77, no. 1 (1972): 15–26, quote 16. This article contains a number of (at least partly) spurious arguments against the validity of the insurance studies' finding that overweight correlates with mortality. For example, Keys and colleagues wrote, "When the relative body weights of persons of various ages are expressed as percentages of desirable or ideal weight, an automatic result is that age and weight are confounded" (24). This criticism lacks relevance since most of the medical-actuarial analyses treated age at issue as a variable, while at least some, such as the Metropolitan study showing improved mortality of overweight people who later lost weight, adjusted expected mortality rates for age. See Louis I. Dublin and Herbert H. Marks,

"Mortality among Insured Overweights in Recent Years," *Transactions of the Association of Life Insurance Medical Directors of America* 35 (1951): 235–263.

19. Of course the actuarial ideal weights derived from them could easily be reexpressed as BMI categories. But BMI could not practically be recalculated and employed as an independent variable in studies based on the insurance data because these older studies would have encoded millions of bits of data on Hollerith-type cards, which would require hand-reordering, repunching, or full reentry in order to perform analyses not originally planned. For comparability, some adjustment based on the average height of the shoes and the weight of the extra clothing and shoes worn in the insurance examinations would also have to be made. On the ascendance of diet-heart, see Ann F. La Berge, "How the Ideology of Low Fat Conquered America," *Journal of the History of Medicine and Allied Sciences* 63, no. 2 (2008): 139–177.

20. Paul Dudley White, "Heart Disease: A Matter of Concern to Executives," *Archives of Environmental Health* 6, no. 3 (1963): 309–311. On Kennedy and hunger abroad, see Nick Cullather, *The Hungry World: America's Cold War Battle against Poverty in Asia* (Cambridge, MA: Harvard University Press, 2013), esp. chap. 5; on domestic hunger in the early 1960s, see Susan Levine, *School Lunch Politics: The Surprising History of America's Favorite Welfare Program* (Princeton, NJ: Princeton University Press, 2011), chap. 6.

21. Poen, *Harry S. Truman versus the Medical Lobby*; Lawrence R. Jacobs, *The Health of Nations: Public Opinion and the Making of American and British Health Policy* (Ithaca, NY: Cornell University Press, 1993), chaps. 7 and 9.

22. Becker, *Outsiders*; Goffman, *Stigma*; Zola, "Medicine as an Institution of Social Control," 487–504; David Frum, *How We Got Here: The 70's: The Decade That Brought You Modern Life (for Better or Worse)* (New York: Basic Books, 2000). Also see Terence Kissack, "Freaking Fag Revolutionaries: New York's Gay Liberation Front, 1969–1971," *Radical History Review* 62 (1995): 105–134; David F. Musto and Pamela Korsmeyer, *The Quest for Drug Control: Politics and Federal Policy in a Period of Increasing Substance Abuse, 1963–1981* (New Haven, CT: Yale University Press, 2002); David T. Courtwright, "The Controlled Substances Act: How a 'Big Tent' Reform Became a Punitive Drug Law," *Drug and Alcohol Dependence* 76, no. 1 (2004): 9–15; Nicolas Rasmussen, *On Speed: The Many Lives of Amphetamine* (New York: New York University Press, 2008), chap. 7.

23. "Curves Have Their Day in Park: 500 at a 'Fat-In' Call for Obesity," *New York Times*, June 5, 1967, 54; Llewellyn Louderback, *Fat Power: Whatever You Weigh Is Right* (New York: Hawthorn, 1970); "Fat Power Wins Chicago Showdown," *Washington Post*, June 11, 1972, A2.

24. Sara G. B. Fishman, "Life in the Fat Underground," *Radiance*, Winter 1998, http://www.radiancemagazine.com/issues/1998/winter_98/fat_underground.html.

25. Sandra Morgen Fishman, *Into Our Own Hands: The Women's Health Movement in the United States, 1969–1990* (New Brunswick, NJ: Rutgers University Press, 2002); Zora Simic, "Fat as a Feminist Issue: A History," in *Fat Sex: New Directions in Theory and Activism*, ed. Helen Hester and Caroline Walters (New York: Routledge, 2016), 15–35.

26. Susie Orbach, *Fat Is a Feminist Issue: The Anti-Diet Guide to Permanent Weight Loss* (New York: Paddington, 1978); Simic, "Fat as a Feminist Issue," 15–35; Marge Dean, *Fat Underground* (Los Angeles, 1979), posted by Charlotte Cooper, August 11, 2016, https://www.youtube.com/watch?v=UPYRZCXjoRo&feature=youtu.be. See especially around the thirty-three-minute mark, where women are exhorted to recognize that their problem is "not because you are oral, and it's not because you're neurotic, or afraid of sex." The problem, they explain, is actually oppression by men.

27. PHS Division of Chronic Disease, Heart Disease Control Program, "Obesity and Health," PHS pub. 1485 (Washington, DC: Government Printing Office, 1966), 2.

28. PHS Division of Chronic Disease, Heart Disease Control Program, "Obesity and Health," 2.

29. PHS Division of Chronic Disease, Heart Disease Control Program, "Obesity and Health," 20–21; see also tables 2 and 3, 8–9.

30. PHS Division of Chronic Disease, Heart Disease Control Program, "Obesity and Health," 23–32, quote 30.

31. PHS Division of Chronic Disease, Heart Disease Control Program, "Obesity and Health," 39–48.

32. PHS Division of Chronic Disease, Heart Disease Control Program, "Obesity and Health," 31, 41.

33. Nathan Hale Jr., *The Rise and Crisis of Psychoanalysis in the United States: Freud and the Americans, 1917–1985* (New York: Oxford University Press, 1995), chaps. 17–20.

34. Susanna McBee, "The End of the Rainbow May Be Tragic: Scandal of the Diet Pills," *Life*, January 26, 1968, 22–29.

35. McBee, "End of the Rainbow," 22–29; "Pill Popping," *Vogue*, November 15, 1969, 104–105; "Diet Pill (Amphetamines) Traffic, Abuse and Regulation," Hearings before the Subcommittee to Investigate Juvenile Delinquency, Senate Committee on the Judiciary, Pursuant to S.Res. 32, sec. 12, 92nd Cong., 1st sess., January 23, 24, 26, 30, 31 and February 2, 1972; "Crime in America—Why 8 Billion Amphetamines?," Hearings of the Select House Committee on Crime, 91st Cong., 1st sess., November 18, 1969; Rasmussen, *On Speed*, chap. 7.

36. William B. Kannel et al., "Relation of Body Weight to Development of Coronary Heart Disease: The Framingham Study," *Circulation* 35 (1967): 734–744.

37. Thomas R. Dawber and William B. Kannel, "Current Status of Coronary Prevention: Lessons from the Framingham Study," *Preventive Medicine* 1, no. 4 (1972): 499–512, quotes 507.

38. T. Gordon and William B. Kannel, "Obesity and Cardiovascular Diseases: The Framingham Study," *Journal of Clinical Endocrinology and Metabolism* 5, no. 2 (1976): 367–375, quote 371.

39. Gordon and Kannel, "Obesity and Cardiovascular Diseases," 367, 371 (estimated), 374–375 (hygienic measure, iconoclasm).

40. It is now widely accepted that adipose tissue contributes to both hypertension and high cholesterol and also (independently) to heart disease, through its metabolic consequences. P. Poirier and R. H. Eckel, "Obesity and Cardiovascular Disease," *Current Atherosclerosis Reports* 4, no. 6 (2002): 448–453; M. Bastien et al., "Overview of Epidemiology and Contribution of Obesity to Cardiovascular Disease," *Progress in Cardiovascular Diseases* 56 (2014): 369–381; P. W. Wilson, "Overweight and Obesity as Determinants of Cardiovascular Risk: The Framingham Experience," *Archives of Internal Medicine* 162 (2002): 1867–1872.

41. Pooling Project Research Group, "Relationship of Blood Pressure, Serum Cholesterol, Smoking Habit, Relative Weight and ECG Abnormalities to Incidence of Major Coronary Events: Final Report of the Pooling Project," *Journal of Chronic Diseases* 31, no. 4 (1978): 201–306. The modest apparent impact of high weight for height, only significant for younger men, was described as an "enigma" (260). A possible explanation is that high risk ratios were not obtained both generally and at older ages because the lowest two weight quintiles of Americans in these studies, with which the top quintiles were compared, included a great many overweight people, especially in their fifties and sixties. This possibility accords with the NHES data.

42. David S. Jones, *Broken Hearts: The Tangled History of Cardiac Care* (Baltimore: Johns Hopkins University Press, 2013), 33–42, 82; Todd M. Olszewski, "The Causal Conundrum: The Diet-Heart Debates and the Management of Uncertainty in American Medicine," *Journal of the History of Medicine and Allied Sciences* 70, no. 2 (2014): 218–249.

43. Veterans Administration Cooperative Study Group, "Effects of Treatment on Morbidity in Hypertension: II. Results in Patients with Diastolic Blood Pressure Averaging 90 through 114 mm Hg," *Journal of the American Medical Association* 213, no. 7 (1970): 1143–1152; Lipid Coronary Primary Prevention Group, "The Lipid Research Clinics Coronary Primary Prevention Trial Results: I. Reduction in Incidence of Coronary Heart Disease," *Journal of the American Medical Association* 251, no. 3 (1984): 351–364; "The Lipid Research Clinics Coronary Primary Prevention Trial Results: II. The Relationship of Reduction in Incidence of Coronary Heart Disease to Cholesterol Lowering," *Journal of the American Medical Association* 251, no. 3 (1984): 365–374.

44. I. D. Frantz et al., "Minnesota Coronary Survey: Effect of Diet on Cardiovascular Events and Deaths" (abstract), *Circulation*, suppl., 52, no. S1 (1975): 4.

45. I. Chalmers, "Underreporting Research Is Scientific Misconduct," *Journal of the American Medical Association* 263, no. 10 (1990): 1405–1408; D. Rennie, "Fair Conduct and Fair Reporting of Clinical Trials," *Journal of the American Medical Association* 282, no. 18 (1999): 1766–1768.

46. Ivan D. Frantz et al., "Test of Effect of Lipid Lowering by Diet on Cardiovascular Risk: The Minnesota Coronary Survey," *Arteriosclerosis, Thrombosis, and Vascular Biology* 9, no. 1 (1989): 129–135, quote 135.

47. C. E. Ramsden et al., "Re-evaluation of the Traditional Diet-Heart Hypothesis: Analysis of Recovered Data from Minnesota Coronary Experiment (1968–73)," *British Medical Journal* 353 (July 2016): 1–17, doi:10.1136/bmj.i1246.

48. As Ramsden et al., "Re-evaluation of the Traditional Diet-Heart Hypothesis," put it, giving the benefit of the doubt to the original researchers' intentions, "One can speculate that the investigators and sponsors would have wanted to distinguish between a failed theory and a failed trial before publication" (13). Keys and Frantz would have known that full publication of their findings would be taken as disproving the diet-heart theory, but they apparently decided that their methodology was too flawed to allow the medical community to draw such a conclusion. Why they did not want medical professionals to reach their own informed decision remains unexplained.

49. Ramsden et al., "Re-evaluation of the Traditional Diet-Heart Hypothesis," i1246; Christopher E. Ramsden et al., "Use of Dietary Linoleic Acid for Secondary Prevention of Coronary Heart Disease and Death: Evaluation of Recovered Data from the Sydney Diet Heart Study and Updated Meta-analysis," *British Medical Journal* 346 (2013): 1–18, doi:10.1136/bmj.e8707. Also see K. Rees et al., " 'Mediterranean' Dietary Pattern for the Primary Prevention of Cardiovascular Disease," *Cochrane Database of Systematic Reviews* 8 (August 2013), doi:10.1002/14651858 .CD009825.pub2.

50. Ancel Keys et al., "The Diet and All-Causes Death Rate in the Seven Countries Study," *Lancet* 8237 (1981): 58–61.

51. American Heart Association, "The Facts on Fats: 50 Years of American Heart Association Dietary Fats Recommendations," June 2015, https://www.heart.org/-/media/files/healthy-living /company-collaboration/inap/fats-white-paper-ucm_475005.pdf, 6;

Ancel Keys and Margeret Keys, *How to Eat Well and Stay Well the Mediterranean Way* (New York: Doubleday 1975); Annie Hubert, "Autour d'un Concept: 'L'alimentation Méditerranéenne,' " *Techniques and Culture* 31–32 (1998): 153–160; Marion Nestle, "Mediterranean Diets: Historical and Research Overview," *American Journal of Clinical Nutrition*, suppl., 61, no. 6 (1995): S1313– S1320; La Berge, "How the Ideology of Low Fat Conquered America," 139–177; Olszewski, "Causal Conundrum," 218–249. WorldCat.org was searched on December 21, 2017, for books with "Mediterranean" as a title word and "cooking" as subject for 1960–1969 and 1970–1979.

52. On dietary recommendations and public acceptance of diets low in saturated fats in the period, see La Berge, "How the Ideology of Low Fat Conquered America," 139–177; Harvey Levenstein, *Paradox of Plenty: A Social History of Eating in Modern America* (Berkeley: University of California Press, 2003), chaps. 11–12; William Rothstein, *Public Health and the Risk Factor: A History of an Uneven Medical Revolution* (Rochester, NY: University of Rochester Press, 2003), 314–321.

53. Hearings before the Select Committee on Nutrition and Human Needs of the United States Senate, "Diet Related to Killer Diseases," July 27–28, 1976 (Washington, DC: Government Printing Office, 1976), 2 (Percy), 7 (Cooper).

54. Hearings before the Select Committee on Nutrition and Human Needs of the United States Senate, "Diet Related to Killer Diseases: II. Part 2," February 1–2, 1977 (Washington, DC: Government Printing Office, 1977). Only one of the four experts who testified, George Cahill of the Joslin Diabetes Center, discussed the physical health consequences of obesity to any extent, and he concentrated on hyperglycemia rather than heart disease. The others dealt with obesity prevention and control.

55. Hearings before the Select Committee on Nutrition and Human Needs of the United States Senate, "Diet Related to Killer Diseases: II. Part 1," February 1–2, 1977 (Washington, DC: Government Printing Office, 1977), Gotto on 316, 321.

56. Hearings before the Select Committee, "Diet Related to Killer Diseases: II. Part 1," Stamler on 294, 299, 301; Levy on 9, 11, 12 (murky).

57. Marion Nestle, *Food Politics: How the Food Industry Influences Nutrition and Health Food* (Berkeley: University of California Press, 2013), 38–43; Gerald M. Oppenheimer and I. Daniel Benrubi, "McGovern's Senate Select Committee on Nutrition and Human Needs versus the Meat Industry on the Diet-Heart Question (1976–1977)," *American Journal of Public Health* 104, no. 1 (2014): 59–69.

58. "Panel Stands by Its Dietary Goals but Eases a View on Eating Meat," *New York Times*, January 24, 1978, 22; "'Dietary Goals' Revision Cooks Up Controversy," *Chicago Tribune*, March 2, 1978, F3; William Rice, "Tug of War over Diet: Nutrition in America Becomes a Political Hot Potato," *Washington Post*, February 9, 1978, E1, E16. The controversy was also discussed in the scientific community; see, for example, Alfred E. Harper, "Dietary Goals: A Skeptical View," *American Journal of Clinical Nutrition* 31, no. 2 (1978): 310–321; D. M. Hegsted, "Dietary Goals: A Progressive View," *American Journal of Clinical Nutrition* 31 (1978): 1504–1509; Jeremiah Stamler, "George Lyman Duff Memorial Lecture: Lifestyles, Major Risk Factors, Proof and Public Policy," *Circulation* 58, no.1 (1978): 3–19; Osmo Turpeinen, "Effect of Cholesterol-Lowering Diet on Mortality from Coronary Heart Disease and Other Causes," *Circulation* 59, no. 1 (1979): 1–7; cf. Oppenheimer and Benrubi, "McGovern's Senate Select Committee on Nutrition and Human Needs," 59–69.

59. Nestle, *Food Politics*; "Dietary Fat Recommendations, 1957–2015," American Heart Association, http://www.heart.org/idc/groups/heart-public/@wcm/@fc/documents/downloadable/ucm _474998.pdf (accessed July 3, 2017); Office of the Surgeon General, US Public Health Service, and Office of the Assistant Secretary for Health, *Healthy People: The Surgeon General's Report on Health Promotion and Disease Prevention*, PHS pub. 79-55071 (Washington, DC: Government Printing Office, 1979), 21, chap. 10.

60. Kent Demaret and Judith Weinraub, "Dr. George Mann Says Low Cholesterol Diets Are Useless, but the 'Heart Mafia' Disagrees," *People*, January 22, 1979, http://people.com/archive/dr -george-mann-says-low-cholesterol-diets-are-useless-but-the-heart-mafia-disagrees-vol-11-no-3.

That the NIH took until 1984 to endorse the diet-heart theory, based on evidence from random-ized controlled trials, may reflect the political pressure on the institution, which prevented action it might have taken earlier based on the preponderance of published evidence. See Office of the Medical Applications of Research, Report of National Heart, Lung, and Blood Institute Consen-sus Conference, "Lowering Blood Cholesterol to Prevent Heart Disease," *Journal of the American Medical Association* 253, no. 14 (1985): 2080–2090.

61. Tavia Gordon and Thomas Thom, "The Recent Decrease in CHD Mortality," *Preventive Medicine* 4, no. 2 (1975): 115–125.

62. Gordon and Thom, "The Recent Decrease in CHD Mortality"; Michael P. Stern, "The Recent Decline in Ischemic Heart Disease Mortality," *Annals of Internal Medicine* 91, no. 4 (1979): 630–640.

63. National Center for Health Statistics, "Anthropometric Reference Data and Prevalence of Overweight, United States, 1976–80," *Vital and Health Statistics*, ser. 11, no. 238 (1987), https://www.cdc.gov/nchs/data/series/sr_11/sr11_238.pdf.

64. H. B. Hubert et al., "Obesity as an Independent Risk Factor for Cardiovascular Disease: A 26-Year Follow-Up of Participants in the Framingham Heart Study," *Circulation* 67, no. 5 (1983): 968–977; William R. Harlan et al., "Secular Trends in Body Mass in the United States, 1960–1980," *American Journal of Epidemiology* 128, no. 5 (1988): 1065–1074.

65. Jeremy Greene, *Prescribing by Numbers: Drugs and the Definition of Disease* (Baltimore: Johns Hopkins University Press, 2006); Rein Vos, *Drugs Looking for Diseases: Innovative Drug Research and the Development of the Beta Blockers and the Calcium Antagonists* (Dordrecht: Springer, 1991); Takuji Hara, *Innovation in the Pharmaceutical Industry: The Process of Drug Dis-covery and Development* (Cheltenham, England: Edward Elgar, 2003); Akira Endo, "A Historical Perspective on the Discovery of Statins," *Proceedings of the Japan Academy*, ser. B, 86, no. 5 (2010): 484–493, doi:10.2183/pjab.86.484.

66. R. J. Kuczmarski et al., "Increasing Prevalence of Overweight among US Adults: The National Health and Nutrition Examination Surveys, 1960 to 1991," *Journal of the American Medical Association* 272, no. 3 (1994): 205–211; K. M. Flegal et al., "Overweight and Obesity in the United States: Prevalence and Trends, 1960–1994," *International Journal of Obesity and Related Metabolic Disorders* 22, no. 1 (1998): 39–47; Cheryl D. Fryar et al., "Prevalence of Overweight, Obesity, and Extreme Obesity among Adults Aged 20 and Over: United States, 1960–1962 through 2013–2014," *National Center for Health Statistics*, July 2016, https://www.cdc.gov/nchs/data/hestat/obesity_adult_13_14/obesity_adult_13_14.pdf.

Index

The letter *f* following a page number indicates a figure.